Five Lectures on the Foundations
of Chinese Medicine

Culture and Knowledge
Edited by Friedrich G. Wallner

Vol. 9

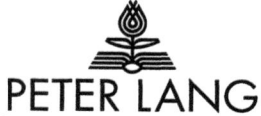

Frankfurt am Main · Berlin · Bern · Bruxelles · New York · Oxford · Wien

Friedrich G. Wallner

Five Lectures on the Foundations of Chinese Medicine

Copyedited by Florian Schmidsberger

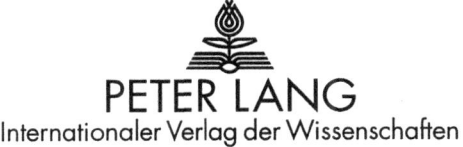

Internationaler Verlag der Wissenschaften

Bibliographic Information published by the Deutsche Nationalbibliothek
The Deutsche Nationalbibliothek lists this publication in the Deutsche Nationalbibliografie; detailed bibliographic data is available in the internet at <http://www.d-nb.de>.

Cover illustration:
„Nike von Samothraki"
Courtesy of Kovac-Verlag.

ISSN 1613-902X
ISBN 978-3-631-57869-8
© Peter Lang GmbH
Internationaler Verlag der Wissenschaften
Frankfurt am Main 2009
All rights reserved.

All parts of this publication are protected by copyright. Any utilisation outside the strict limits of the copyright law, without the permission of the publisher, is forbidden and liable to prosecution. This applies in particular to reproductions, translations, microfilming, and storage and processing in electronic retrieval systems.

www.peterlang.de

Dedicated to my friends
in the Basic Theory Institute
of China Academy for Chinese Medical Sciences

Table of Content

I. Introduction 9

1. Fritz Wallner: The Theoretical Structure and Methodology of TCM 11
2. Kurt Greiner, Fritz Wallner: Innovative Ontology and Methodology: An Introduction into Constructive Realism (CR) 17

II. Five Lectures on the Foundations of Chinese Medicine .. 25

1. Fritz Wallner: The comparison between Western medicine and TCM 27
2. Fritz Wallner: Advantages of TCM 35
3. Fritz Wallner: The research method in medicine 41
4. Fritz Wallner: How to establish an integrative medicine? 49
5. Fritz Wallner: Modernization of TCM without Westernization 55

III. Extension: Contribution of other TCM scientists 61

1. Zhang Weibo: Strangification of TCM by Western Science: Under Which Conditions can Western Science be used in TCM Correctly? 63
2. Lan Feng-Li: Globalization of TCM: Cultural Differences between TCM and Western Medicine 77
3. Günter Gunia: Development and Possibilities of TCM 95

I. Introduction

1. FRITZ WALLNER: THE THEORETICAL STRUCTURE AND METHODOLOGY OF TCM

Presentation of the Research Project in the occasion of the opening of the SINO-AUSTRIAN-Research-Institute
17th September 2007

1.1. Introduction

It is a special pleasure for me to speak here as I already did a lot of research on Traditional Chinese Medicine (TCM). As well I have planed to do a lot of further research on TCM in the next 10 years. We can say that there will be a big jump for the theoretical structure and methodology of TCM in the next 4 years. This presentation contains 4 chapters:
1. First I want to introduce our research group.
2. Then I will state our comprehension of TCM.
3. Then I will present the research programme we elaborated.
4. Probably the most interesting part: I will show the service that is offered to Western science with this research – especially pharmacology.

1.2. Introduction of our TCM-research group

1) *Professor Fritz G. Wallner*: I do not want to say many things about me. I am Professor for philosophy of science at Vienna University. I started as a specialist for the so called "Vienna Circle". I modified the ideas of the Vienna Circle because of

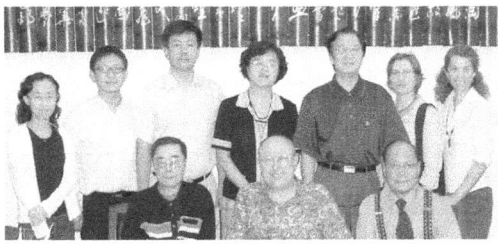

Illustration 1: TCM research group

the unsolved problems. By concentrating on the unsolved problems of the Vienna Circle I developed a new philosophy of science: the position of the so called *"Constructive Realism"*. The Constructive Realism – as I recognised later – is very helpful to make the specific structure of TCM understandable. Until now I have been researching TCM for nineteen years. Since 1994 I offer a seminar in the Vienna University on traditional Chinese medicine every year.

2) *Dr. Guijuan Pan*: I also want to introduce my colleague. We both are in the chair of the research group: She is the dean of China academy of Chinese

Medical Sciences. She is a top scientist studying TCM for 20 years. She was able to get the highest level fund from the Chinese Government, the 973-fund for a very special project. She gives us the possibility to make a real deep view into the structure of TCM. We both have published a lot of books and papers. We are cooperating with a lot of different TCM-universities and colleges in China like TCM-University of Shanghai, TCM-University of Yunnan, TCM-University of Harbin and so on.

3) *Other scientists*: We also have other scientists from other TCM-Universities like *Prof. Zhi-Zhong Li* from the Hong Kong Baptist University. Then *Prof. Lu Guangxin* from the China Academy of Chinese medical sciences in Beijing. Some of them are not present in the picture for instance *Prof. Zhu Ming* from the University of TCM in Beijing and some others. I cannot mention all.

1.3. Our comprehension of TCM

If we have a look to the *Dao*, the *Jing*, the *Qi* and the *Shen* you see one thing. It is impossible to make a corresponding relation between the Western thinking and TCM. Because *Dao* is not just a methodology. *Dao* is also ontology. And *Jing* is not essence. Jing is a lot. Also be careful with *Qi*. Everybody says Qi is energy. But this is nonsense. Shen is another important problem. I name these just to introduce how far we are away to understand the TCM completely in the present. The main problem is: if you really want to do a research in TCM, you have to become aware at first that there are *differences between Western medicine and TCM* that make them *incommensurable*.

Let us talk about the incommensurability of Western medicine and TCM: To explain and to show the incommensurability of TCM and Western medicine I want to express four essential aspects:

Differences	WM	TCM
1. Methodological	induction and deduction	Qu Xiang Bi Lei
2. Ontological	analysis/ synthesis/ abstraction	leaves all as it is
3. Experience	reducing the subject	unification of subject and object
4. Theoretical structure	rules and laws	pattern recognition and interpretation

Table 1: Incommensurability of WM and TCM

– *Methodology*: If you consider the methodology in the Western medicine, you find the concepts of *induction* and *deduction* – while in TCM not. The most important method of TCM – *Qu Xiang Bi Lei* – is related to phenomena. It is similar to the core of the position of phenomenology: to go back to the things. The named method aims that the things are coming with themselves instead of using abstractions and concepts which are not illustrative. For example when the TCM doctor speaks about a "heat in the liver". This is another world of thinking. Who does not understand this should keep silent because he doesn't understand anything.

- *Ontology*: I want to mention this aspect because for Europeans it is so hard to understand that there is another system which has the claim of truth and a system takes a different way as we do in our thinking. In the Western way of thinking you find ontological analysis/synthesis/abstraction. Instead TCM leaves all as it is.
- *Experience*: It is the Western way of thinking to *reduce the subject* in scientific work. It is the claim to take out your subjectivity from the object. Instead the Chinese way of thinking is based on a *unification of the subject and object*.
- *Theoretical structure*: In Western science we know *rules and laws*. Chinese science works with *pattern recognition and interpretation*. Interpretation is very important. The Chinese characters are some reality for the research. This is a point we have to a lot of research in the next years.

In Short: you cannot understand a book if you just check the letters. It is the same, if you just look for TCM with the methods of Western medicine. In this case you will not be able to understand this system of medicine. So it is important to *take care of the approach*.

1.4. Our research programme

The necessity for a TCM-adequate research: Let us focus on the following essential question: What does an adequate research in TCM have to do? What should it be like? I now want to present a program for research for the following four years.

1) *Semantical analysis of the concepts*: It is quite unclear what is "fire" or "metal" or "wood" in TCM. This is not as we say in English or German. This has a different meaning. Fire is an interesting point for a semantical analysis for instance. And wood is nothing which is ontological. Wood has a metaphorical sense. Wood expresses that all is growing. Therefore all translations in English and German books are wrong.
2) *Syntactical analysis of the sentences*: In the Nei Jing – let me say the bible for TCM-people – you have sentences which are not just describing. This is the big difference to the Western science.
3) *Qu Xiang Bi Lei* – following the circular reasoning by phenomena: This is one point: Everybody who wants to tell us something about TCM has to be familiar with this method. Before you are not able to use this method your statements about TCM are deficient.

The detailed contents of the project:
1) *The comparison between Western medicine & TCM*: As an example let us think of the ways how the Western and the traditional Chinese medicine understand the human body. In the Western world you will find anatomic pictures that illustrate the single organs in the human body as well as their positions. If you look at the illustrations of TCM they show you a human body that is not opened with scalpels. On these pictures you can see the different meridians. It should be evident that there is no direct comparison possible. There is a very important question: What are the meridians? This is already a big topic of questions; it is a big question to understand this system. But this has nothing to do with neurology as you can read in some books.
2) *Culture and Philosophy in TCM*: We also have to emphasize on the aspect of culture and philosophy in TCM. Let us consider some elements of its philosophy: For example the Yin-Yang-Symbol. You know that all is contained in the Yin. Yin is in the Yang and the Yang is in the Yin. Let us also think of the Wu Xing. The Wu Xing is an interesting thing in the history of understanding TCM in the Western world. In most of the books you can read five elements – but this is wrong. Sometimes you even can read that you can compare it with the old Greek medicine as they had similar elements – but this is nonsense.

It would be more precise, if we said "five basis of changing". Because the matter wood and earth and so on correspond to movements, to a specific type of movement. Wood corresponds to growing, earth corresponds to balance. – These are our first approaches. I do not say that I know. I just know a little bit about this. We have to do a lot of studies to come closer to this thinking.
3) *The methodology of TCM and clinical practice*: Let us think of a certain Chinese symbol, the "Yellow Emperor's Inner Classics" (Illustration 2: Chinese character). I should explain this character: originally it means – as my friend told me – "viewpoints". We have to do this as methodology. Here you can see again the big difficulties we have. We have to give the characters a new interpretation. At the end of my lecture I will show you how we have to deal with methods from the Western world to do this.

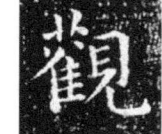

Illustration 2: Chinese character

4) *The basic concepts of TCM theory*: Let us refer to the idea of the Qi. This is just a metaphor – just to make this clear. This is a system which is used in the Qi Gong-Theory. Here we have different places. The place for the Nau (the brain) or the place for the Qin (the heart) or the place for Shen and so on. You must not think that the position of the organs has any meaning for TCM. The locality is without any importance. It is important that they make a construction which is using the function of the organs in the system of TCM. The function of the organs gives them a place in the system. If they say here

is Xin (heart) or here is Nao (brain) and so on, they want to tell us that this is just a metaphor about the cooperation of these organs. Again: it is a main point of understanding TCM that we understand that the organs have just a function. They don't tell us something what we would call "ontological".
5) *The correct English translation of TCM-texts*: I think this is a very high aim but we are convinced to reach it. But we only can do it as long as we understand it. Therefore it will be a long way. It is clear that it does not make sense to translate specific terms of TCM into English or German. You have to keep the Chinese word and explain the Chinese word in a type of dictionary by paraphrasing it. Then you can give the reader and the Western doctor an impression what this term means in its original sense.

1.5. Service offer for Western science

1) *Different information in respect to the body from different point of view*: Our service for Western science has two aspects: The first aspect is the easier one: We offer information of the body, information of medicine which is incompatible to the information you have.

   The first consideration is that it is necessary for the Westerner in pharmacology or medicine that he becomes aware: here is a system which explains diseases, which explains different ways of the body in a different way. You can act – I think – as a Westerner in this way that you say: on the one side we have the one, the old universe, while on the other side we have the new universe – so you have two universes. Sometimes we have to change from the one to the other one. But clearly this is not satisfying at the end.

2) *Take care of relativity – Strangification*: Therefore I want to introduce a methodology of philosophy of science which I have found myself more than 10 years ago for other questions. It is able to make a combination of both. But it is surprising like a child is surprised. You will enter a new world, if you use this. In the Western philosophy of science this methodology is named Strangification, in German "Verfremdung". It names the experience you get, if you come into a different context. Then these things you want to say or you thought are somehow mirrors in this different context. You can see the presuppositions of your own ideas.

   I want to give you an example. For instance take the concept of "blood pressure". High blood pressure is an important disease for Westerners. In TCM you have different explanations, elaborated ones. For instance heat in the liver combined with restricted liver-Qi can be one cause of blood pressure. There are other causes, too. Therefore if you look for pharmaca, first take a look what they mean for Chinese medicine. But don't just take a look for a pharmacon which takes away the high blood pressure – this is Western style. This is a different way. Therefore this is our offer to the Western pharmacology: You will learn a lot. You can do so much if you are able to understand this theory.

To give you another example: Gastritis corresponds to five different diseases in Chinese medicine. By pharmacology – if you understand the Chinese medicine – you must treat everyone of this disease *in a different way*. This is an important difference which you have to learn to understand if you really want to make pharmacology for TCM. And this does not mean just to touch the surface and take something which is useful for us. It would be a pity, if we lose this elaborated system of the old Chinese times which is really scientific. Believe me, it is a long time of research I have been doing the last years.

2. KURT GREINER, FRITZ WALLNER: INNOVATIVE ONTOLOGY AND METHODOLOGY: AN INTRODUCTION INTO CONSTRUCTIVE REALISM (CR)

2.1. Preliminary remark

The philosophical system of the Viennese School of Constructive Realism offers an innovative ontology as well as a new epistemology. Both concepts can be used as methodological basic tools by modern scientists of the 21st century. Before we start to reconstruct the development of the ontological and epistemological innovations of Constructive Realism we look back on the historical situation when we have started our epistemological work in the end of the 20th century.
In the late 1980th and the early 1990th we entered scientific laboratories for the first time and we took the chance to observe what scientists actually were doing. We recognized very quickly that the scientific doing is a complex set of different activities but it has nothing to do with the "description of the world". It is no searching for truth or something like this. The everyday job of the natural scientist is the building of constructions by means of certain data and specific information. Scientists put different data and information into a constructed framework and feed it into the computer to check what is possible within this framework, to check which data are ordered within this framework and which are not. This is constructive acting by data management but there is no description.

Construction and comprehension instead of description and metaphysical truth

In those times we asked: What do scientists intend with their constructions besides their instrumentalist aims? We were interested in their specific desires when they were working in their laboratories in the departments of physics, biology etc. Finally we found out that their real desire is to understand the results of their own productions. In general scientists want to understand what the results of their constructions mean. Their intention is comprehension and not to find metaphysical truth. Truth of the ontological laws of the given world is just ideology. The argument of scientific struggling for truth is interesting for politicians and can be used to make money. However, the outcome of our personal discussions with working scientists shows that scientists first of all are interested in understanding their own activities because they are just able to handle with their specific system of formal propositions but they do not know what the given construction and the system of propositions really mean. Indeed, if working scientists should attempt to translate their proposition system into normal everyday language they would have encounter difficulties and would not know how to do this.

The results of our experiences and investigations in the filed of working scientists firstly pointed out the necessity to substitute the claim of description by the phenomenon of construction and secondly showed the priority of comprehensibility instead of the classical scientific claim of legitimation. Now the main question was how understanding of scientific activities of construction can be reached. To find an answer it was necessary to work out an innovative system of ontological thinking. That means at first it was necessary to invent a new philosophical perspective on the "given world", the "scientific reality" ("micro-worlds") and the "cultural context" which then could be used as a basis for developing a specific epistemological methodology.

2.2. An Innovative Ontology in Constructive Realism: The Difference between "Given World", "Scientific Reality" / "Micro-Worlds" and "Cultural Context"

With the development of our constructive realistic system we have created philosophy of science *for* scientists and even not philosophy of science *about* science or scientists. In our contemporary situation it is important that scientists are able to see the necessity of our constructive realistic intentions. It is important for them to recognize that a completely new and different philosophical framework becomes necessary. Today a philosophy of science must be able to support scientists with their efforts to understand what scientific construction is if scientists want to protect the classical claim of European science called "Erkenntnis" (knowledge).

About the given world

We are convinced that scientific constructions are *real* although the constructive procedure is *fictive*. Constructions are fictive in the sense that we are able to construct different versions of worlds in our mind, for example a world of love or a world of war or a world of whatever. This is fiction of course. But at the same time the fictive procedure of build up scientific constructions become real in the specific sense that we are able to act and work with them for scientific purposes. That means that if we are successful in achieving special aims by using specific scientific constructions than they become reality. If we successfully devise a scientific proposition system in the direction of technology the world will be changed. Scientific constructions change the world and react in some way. In every instance the "given world" (*Wirklichkeit*) or what we call "nature" is changed by the successful realization of a scientific proposition system.

We can already see that constructivist ontology in the context of Constructive Realism is not understood in the classical metaphysic sense, not as a description of the deep structures of the given world but rather as an instrument which helps scientists to avoid categorical mistakes. Constructive Realists make a strict distinction between the "given world" and what scientists actually describe with their scientific activities.

Of course you can change nature in your mind or you can change nature in reality. Changing nature in the mind is the forerunner of changing nature in reality. In the case of medicine for example you will treat the body in totally different ways whether you apply Chinese medicine or European medicine. In both constructions you change nature because you do not handle the real body you just handle the cultural determined image of the body. Let us repeat: Science does not describe the true structure of the given world and so neither Chinese medicine nor European medicine describes the real body. Both of them make use of a construction of the body which creates relations between different parts of the body inside the body, relations which create theories of functioning with respect to the body. In constructive realistic perspective the sum of all these cultural dependent different constructions *replaces* the given world. If we go to a doctor and tell him about our problem, the European doctor will react totally differently in comparison to the Chinese doctor. You have the same body in both cases but the European doctor will come up with a theory maybe connected with something such as urine and the Chinese doctor will also come up with a theory which might be connected with different forces in the body.

It is important to see that scientists of course cannot describe the given world or nature but rather artificial products that have been created through abstractions from the "cultural context" (life-world / *Lebenswelt*) of human beings, from their experiences of nature.

About scientific reality and its micro-worlds

For scientists the meaning of the term "reality" usually is completely clear but reality sometimes causes difficulties for philosophers. Reality in our constructive realistic context is only understood in the way that proposition systems of science build a specific world or an imago of the world which can *partly replace* or *substitute* the given world. Exactly in this special sense science has to do with reality. This world which is created and built up by scientific constructions is that world Constructive Realists call "scientific reality" (*Realität*).

Scientific constructions are clearly constructions of materials taken from experience and used for technical reasons. In a scientific laboratory for example you gather much information by a lot of data. People having good ideas in formal languages, in mathematics, in mathematical models or in models created by mathematicians become able to structure this information. One structure for specific information might be better, another structure might be worse. These scientific structures are made for achieving specific goals. Therefore if you use your structure for a specific set of information you are not explicitly defining your goals but you at least intimate a definition. Here you may be confronted with several questions: What do you want to show by means of this structure? Which prognoses can you make by means of it? What is not excluded by this structure? What is not possible by means of this structure?

Scientific reality is the world which we handle by means of science. The scientific propositions describe this type of an artificial world. Single Scientific propositions (re)produced in various scientific fields are those reality-aspects Constructive Realists call "micro-worlds" (*Mikrowelten*). Micro-worlds do not describe nature, they describe produced reality. They describe how to handle the world with which we are dealing. For reasons of terminology and of clearness we must differentiate between scientific realities because scientific reality changes. Scientific reality in our times is not the same as scientific reality was in the 19th century and scientific reality of the next century will be different to that with which we are acting now. Scientific reality depends on various cultural, social, historical and scientific situations.

A famous proponent of this view on scientific activities beside Constructive Realism is the constructivist philosophy of science supported by the "School of Erlangen" arguing that modern physicists (apart from few exceptions) don't share the naive-realistic correspondence theory of truth. Science as an activity of producing knowledge is not loaded with the claim that the results of this knowledge production are the so called "natural laws" as a fix representation of the one and homogenous reality. On the contrary, current physicists deal with self-produced constructions and not with objects existing without human actions that can't be thus discovered. Physicists are no longer naturalists deciphering the world and its code, but according to this view and self-understanding their core task is making technology possible. Modern physics don't draw the divine construction plan of the world-machine, but rather generate knowledge (scientific reality / micro-worlds) that allows constructing machines to facilitate our life.

About the cultural context or life-world

If we look again on our distinction between the "given world" which cannot be recognized on the one hand and the "scientific reality" respectively "micro-worlds" which are totally constructed by scientists on the other hand we will certainly get into contact with the following metaphysical question: Should we doubt that the given world exists?

Constructive Realists cannot find a good reason to doubt that the given world exists. According to Wittgenstein we do not doubt the existence of the given world. Consequently we should not discuss this doubt about the existence of the given world. Instead of the term "given world" we can also say "environment". Because the given world in our descriptive system is the world with which we are living. The given world is not the world of our intellectual ambitions, the given world is the world which supports our own existence.

Even Constructive Realism differentiates between the world which is established by constructions called scientific reality and the given world they cannot find a reason to doubt about the existence of a world which is actually not constructed. However we cannot say anything about this world because all our discussion about world is guided by constructing. Constructing leads to discussion and enables us to describe something. Without constructing there would be no description. Therefore, in addition to scientific reality, we must assume that there is a non-constructed world which we cannot describe. This given world or environment has the function to support, to guide and to enable our life-process.

According to these considerations we can define environment as all that is beyond knowledge but nevertheless strongly connected with our lives. Environmental processes are processes outside processes of knowledge and cognition. Knowledge processes are different to environmental processes. Because of this reason we have to distinguish the constructive realistic division between environment and scientific reality from Immanuel Kant's division between the world of the senses and the object in itself.

If you consider the difference between scientific reality and environment and the fact that scientific reality is connected with scientific knowledge then it will become clear that there is something which is not scientific knowledge but also a type of knowledge based on cultural foundation – the knowledge of everyday life. All the various types of knowledge in the context of life world are introduced by specific cultural backgrounds and clearly these types of knowledge are different in different cultures. "Life world" or "cultural context" (*Lebenswelt*) in Constructive Realism simply means all the types of knowledge which guide and manage our everyday lives for achieving our existential goals. Life world knowledge is introduced by cultural education and training which are not reflected in a scientific way. But of course life world knowledge influences the construction of scientific reality. In this fact we can find the reason why each kind of scientific reality (including all various types of micro-worlds) depends on its cultural background because the cultural context is always the basis on which scientific reality can be developed. In other words: No science without culture!

2.3. An Innovative Methodology in Constructive Realism: The Hermeneutical Technique of "Strangification"

From the constructivist viewpoint of philosophy of science the instrumentalistic dimension of science is not problematic, but what is problematic in sciences is its self-reflexive dimension. That's why we will deal with the issue of a technique of understanding that is relevant to understanding, and not with the issue of technology that is relevant to actions. Or, in other words, we will discuss the issue of knowledge, or more exactly, of self-knowledge.

Communication in interdisciplinary teams and its function for self-knowledge

According to the constructive-realistic perspective it is a fact that scientists are not able to recognise what they do in the course of micro-world construction. Enclosed in their scientific language games (Wittgenstein) it is not possible to obtain the necessary distance to this language game, and without distance it isn't possible to achieve knowledge.
Standing on our foundation of a completely reformed ontological theory we can ask again: how can scientific activities of construction be understood?
Looking back in the early 1990th when we organized epistemological teams where specialists from physics, biology, sociology, history etc. had the chance for interdisciplinary discussions we found the answer in a curious way. During a discussion-seminar about a particular problem of one science we had the experience that it was terribly difficult for a physicist to find a language which is understandable even for people from biology, sociology or history. In this situation we had the experience that if a physicist is able to make his proposition system understandable to those coming from other scientific fields he will be able to understand his own proposition system in a much better way after this presentation. This means that when he is able to explain his proposition system to his colleagues from other fields in everyday language he is at the same time able to understand his own actions, his own scientific working.

Understanding the own proposition system by the help of strangification

As a consequence Constructive Realists have developed a hermeneutical technique of understanding called "strangification" (*Verfremdung*) claiming to take a proposition system X out of its original context K and to place in another context R. This method causes the scientist to place his theory in a different and strange context. From the viewpoint of this context R the theory X is considered, assessed, etc. newly and, that's for sure, differently. Strangification means hence to leave the ways of thinking of a special discipline. Without referring to any meta-theoretical instances the procedure of strangification reveals implicit pre-

requisites of a theory unknown and unrecognised by scientists before strangification. Mostly strangification gives rise to a relativation of the original theory. Strangification opens a new understanding of a scientific method – insights that wouldn't be disclosed in the manner of instrumentalist work.
Strangification as a methodological procedure by which you take a proposition system (a system of presuppositions) out of its original context and put it into a strange context means for example: transfer the proposition system of elementary physics to sociology or transfer the proposition system of Traditional Chinese Medicine to Western Medicine and have a look at what will happen.
The first impression usually is that this proposition system becomes totally arbitrary because there are no terms for it in other languages. There are elements which must be given new names in the terminology which is understandable for those from the strange discipline. At first it is very difficult for a physicist to abandon his way of thinking. He must somehow liberate himself from his own science. Once he achieves this he becomes understandable and suddenly he is able to understand his own proposition system in a much better way than before. Consequently strangification means to transfer a proposition system into a totally different context for discussing it with others. In this way scientists become able to understand the structure of their own proposition system.

The translational structure of strangification

The reason for these effects can be found in the philosophical system of Ludwig Wittgenstein. Wittgenstein explains that every kind of language is an activity which makes a lot of presuppositions. Language between two or more people only functions if they are able and willing to understand each other's presuppositions. It is not enough to learn a strange language it is also necessary to understand the implicit presuppositions of the other language. This is intimate knowledge. Therefore if you translate your proposition system into another context the presuppositions become visible. It becomes clear what a scientist presupposes if he takes his specific proposition system out of its original scientific context.
This is a similar procedure as in the real situation of translation. For example if you translate from Chinese into German you will surely learn a lot about presuppositions of the Chinese language which you cannot recognize if you just speak Chinese language. When you perform a translation you can see what you are not able to express in the other language, you can see which tools the other language has which are not used in your language.
And in the same structural way the method of strangification functions especially for scientific purposes. According to these basic principles strangification has a self-reflection motivating and knowledge encouraging effect on microworld constructors. Finally strangification is an instrument or tool that leads to scientific understanding and knowledge.

2.4. Final considerations

If we look on the situation of sciences in the 21st century we have to state that systematic reflection is an indispensably condition for scientific work. If the procedure of constructing and (re)producing micro-worlds is not reflected scientific reality would lose its scientific importance, it would lose its role and its function for scientific knowledge. Especially reflection on scientific reality by the methodological help of the constructive realistic technique of strangification is absolutely necessary if we want to protect the classical European claim of science (*Erkenntnis*) as we know it.

2.5. Literature

Greiner, Kurt; Wallner, Fritz (Hg.): *Konstruktion und Erziehung. Zum Verhältnis von konstruktivistischem Denken und pädagogischen Intentionen.* Hamburg: Verlag Dr. Kovac 2003.

Greiner, Kurt: *Therapie der Wissenschaft. Eine Einführung in die Methodik des Konstruktiven Realismus.* Frankfurt: Peter Lang 2005.

Wallner, Fritz: *Wissenschaft in Reflexion.* Wien: Braumüller Verlag 1992.

Wallner, F.: *Konstruktion der Realität. Von Wittgenstein zum Konstruktiven Realismus.* Wien: WUV Universitätsverlag 1992.

Wallner, F.: A*cht Vorlesungen über den Konstruktiven Realismus.* Wien: WUV Universitätsverlag 1992.

Wallner, F.: Die *Verwandlung der Wissenschaft. Vorlesungen zur Jahrtausendwende.* Hrsg. v. M. J. Jandl. Hamburg: Verlag Dr. Kovac 2002.

II. Five Lectures on the Foundations of Chinese Medicine

1. FRITZ WALLNER: THE COMPARISON BETWEEN WESTERN MEDICINE AND TCM

1st lecture at the China Academy of Chinese Medical Sciences in Beijing
7th September 2007

1.1. Introduction: about the analysis of the scientific and theoretical structure of TCM

I want to begin this lecture with 3 questions:
1. China has a lot of different sciences: astronomy, physics, chemistry and also medicine. Why didn't these sciences survive beside medicine?
2. Why did the traditional Chinese medicine survive?
3. What are the advantages of the Chinese medicine?

Let me try to answer these questions:

ad 1. Chinese sciences – except its medicine – did not survive because they did not take care enough about ontology and methodology. The success of Western science is based on its reasoning that focuses on *ontology* and *methodology*. In the Western world it started in the time of old Greek.

ad 2. Chinese medicine has the advantage that – compared to the ontology of Western medicine – its thinking is more adequate to the course of life, to the structure of living systems. The Western ontology is directed to dead things. The Western ontology did not take care enough about living systems. During this lecture you will hear a lot of information about this.

ad 3. I am going to answer the third question more detailed in my second lecture that has the title "advantages of TCM"[1].

There are two reasons to study the scientific, the theoretical structure of TCM. – The first reason is an external one. You have to discuss, you have to cooperate, and somehow you have to survive *beside* Western medicine and also *with* Western medicine. Therefore you need to have arguments for this discussion. It is important to protect the discussion about the scientific, about the theoretical structure against a wrong approach from the Western world.

The second reason is even more important. The second reason deals with a very important contemporary tendency you can find nearly everywhere in China: "modernization" – for example: "Modernization of TCM". This is really important. But modernization should be done in the right way – it should be a modernization *without losing* the *concept*, the *idea* or the *structure of TCM* – instead

---

[1] See "Fritz Wallner: Advantages of TCM", page 35.

of understanding modernization as an *adaptation to Western science.* – This is also the main reason for these series of lectures in September: *that you and we together learn how to research TCM in an adequate way.*
This lecture is divided into 3 chapters:
1. The first chapter has the title: *What can we expect from science?*
2. The second: The framework of *comparison between TCM and Western medicine.*
3. The third one: *the cultural conditions of science.*

1.2. What can we expect from science?

Science is a procedure that enables you to get a survey, to get an understandable explanation. – This is a more general definition of science than the traditional one. The traditional definition of science was depending on the traditional European idea about ontology and causality and so on. But in the last 30 years it became clear that these ideas are problematic. Therefore – as we will see during the lecture – this definition covers both the Western science and the traditional Chinese medicine. Because it was clearly nonsense to say Western medicine is *science* and Chinese medicine is *culture – both are cultures*. Western medicine is culture in Europe; Chinese medicine is culture of China. To understand this definition of science we have to look to the differences between the Western science and the Chinese science.

I want to refer to three important contemporary philosophers from the field of philosophy of science: Karl Popper, Kurt Gödel and Thomas Kuhn. Every one of them did a lot of reform in the Western science. Unfortunately there is no time to discuss here in detail. I just want to point out that the structure of Western science *is difference* to the structure of TCM.

In the Western science it is important to make a *combination of experience and logics.* For Chinese science experiences are also important but in another sense while logic has another structure. There is logic in Chinese science, but you cannot compare these logics to Western logics. To make this argument clearer and more understandable I want to state two examples: Take a look at the kidney deficiencies in TCM. We take three examples to show symptoms that are connected to deficiencies of kidneys: loss of hair, amnesia, soreness of waist. There are *different manifestations at different persons*. After that we want to take a look at the different situation and the different way of Western medicine. As an example we take bacteria infection. Bacteria infection can lead to pneumonia for instance and has the *same manifestation at different persons*.

But here you have to be careful. Here is one crucial point of understanding. The relation between the bacteria in the pneumonia is not the same relation as the relation between kidney deficiencies, loss of hair and so on. In the Western medicine it is thought that this relation is causal, a way of *causal connection. You must not take this idea to understand TCM.* The connection between kidney

deficiency and loss of hair and so on is *not causal*. I will tell you in the last part of this lecture more about this relation. But keep in mind: *It is not causal*.
From these examples we can learn that it is not necessary to expect explanation by causality from science. I do not want that you suffer and you ask about the relation of Chinese science. Therefore I give you just a short hint: The relation is a *type of phenomenology*. But anyway, keep in mind again that science can be understood in different ways: by making causal relation and by using with other tools and other ways.

1.3. The framework of comparison between TCM and Western medicine

Until now you should understand: To be able to compare TCM and Western medicine it is necessary to have a fitting and adequate framework. If you think of the framework of Western medicine, you will lose the structure of TCM. Therefore we have to invent a framework *that covers both Western medicine and TCM*. Therefore we have to go away from the traditional thinking of ontology and methodology of the Western world. I want to give you a hint: If a Westerner gets results in his scientific research, he believes that this is a *description of nature*. But this is a wrong idea. We have to find concepts that take care of Western medicine and TCM as well. About twenty years ago I invented a position in the field of philosophy of science that offers an ontology that fits for both medical systems. We named it "Constructive Realism".

I want to explain this ontology in a simple way: Ontology is the *approach to the world*. For both medical systems we have an approach to the world that divides two aspects of the world. The one aspect we name "actuality" – what is given. To give you an example from medicine: pain for instance is given. You cannot describe it. But you can describe the character of pain to or you can give an explanation of pain. It means that we have to conceptualize the pain and then we get another aspect, another shape of the world – and this shape we name "reality". Therefore you can understand first that *reality* is *another level* of the world than *actuality*. In the Western medicine a disease is reality. We name every disease a "micro-world". We also can name a system of diseases a micro-world. You may now understand that the sum of micro worlds is the reality for specific human being, for a specific culture, for a specific situation in history and so on. Therefore the Westerner has another reality than the Chinese people. Probably they have the same actuality.

You know that the concept of diseases in TCM is different from Western medicine. We can even say in a strict sense: *In TCM there are no diseases or TCM is not directed to diseases*. We can learn from this consideration that different micro-worlds are *independent of each other*. There is one essential point you really have to take care of: *you cannot mix these two micro-worlds*. For example: you cannot blend the micro-world of the Western medicine and the micro-world of the meridian. So you cannot say meridians are like the neural system. This is nonsense. The comparison cannot be done directly. Instead the comparison has to go to the presuppositions of these systems. We will speak about these presuppositions in the last chapter.

I would like to underline that the main research in the future has to focus on this question: *What are the ontological implications of the meridian system* and *what are the ontological implications of the Western medicine?* Because you now understand an essential aspect: *They have different ontological presuppositions.* I give you an example: Two days before I found an article by one of your colleagues. He pointed out that acupuncture cannot be done without relation to Shen. Therefore you may understand: *if you do acupuncture just in the Western way, you are misleading.*

Let us take a look at the question how we get experience. We have to be aware that experience is *always a construct with a content which is structured by concepts.* Therefore you already understand on this level that experience in TCM *cannot be the same* as experience in the Western medicine. – But there is an additional strong argument I will tell you in the next chapter. Considering these examples the microscope is *not* the *"better eye"*, the microscope is *another way to look.* If you use microscopes, you lose some aspects that you only can get, if you look without any additional instruments. Every one in a laboratory is working with it.

Based on this consideration it is easy to go to a result which is always strange for the Westerners. Traditional Chinese medicine and Western medicine get *two different diagnoses.* As a consequence you cannot compare both in the way that you say that the diagnosis in TCM is the same as in Western medicine. Therefore a direct comparison, a direct combination of both medical systems is misleading and as a result you would lose the original structure of TCM. If you for instance take concepts of the Western medicine into the system of TCM, you will destroy the TCM.

1.4. Cultural conditions

I give you a hint in cultural studying: If Western medicine and TCM are connected directly, Western medicine will not win because it was better or more true, but because of the cultural background: The cultural background of Western medicine is the culture of Europe and its culture has an aggressive aspect because it has the statement that there is *only one truth, only one explanation* – like only one God. Compared to Chinese people it is very easy to understand that there are *different ways of truth* – for Westerners this is very hard to accept.

Let us go to the cultural conditions of science. If we for example think of the religious buildings of both cultures, you will see that there are different understandings of ways to live. If you are living in this way or if you are praying in another way, both ways offer different ways of understanding life. In science scientific knowledge always starts with the wide world, with the every day problems. You also can find this aspect in the history of Western science and you see it clearly in TCM. Therefore science always has the *background of different cultural convictions*.

1.4.1. Cultural conditions of Western science

Let us look to the cultural conditions of Western medicine. The Western medicine presupposes concepts that are fundamental for all Western sciences: for example the *strict division between subject and object*. But everybody knows that this is an ideal goal that cannot be reached. But as a scientist in the Western world or as a scientist in Western science – today also Western science is common in China – you always have to be aware to take out usual aspects from your scientific work.

I want to give you an example from my own experience. It refers to everyday life of university. If I for instance recommend somebody in my university, I have to be aware that I strictly take out all personal aspects. If I said, he is a good friend, he won't be taken. In China this is an argument for taking him because if I say, someone special was a good friend of mine they are happy that I know him and they will take him. – Different views. Both views are somehow good and somehow bad.

The Westerner way of thinking is the way of *induction and deduction*. Induction is the way from the single case to the general, to the more general case and to the universal theory at the end. Deduction is the way from the theory to the single cases. You can imagine its influence for medicine. Therefore it is a problem of university's education in medicine in the Western world that the doctors have to learn real medicine, if they complete university.

Let us consider three important European philosophers: *Tales, Plato, Aristotle*. We can learn from them something about the way we should work together – if you want – in the next years. We could learn from them something about our cooperation, for our research in the next years. To do this we should take care of their positions and their differences: Tales started *to develop science*. Plato elaborated a big *system of ontology*. Aristotle elaborated a *system of methodology*. Therefore what we can learn is not just to make science but always to be aware about the relation of science and the world – *ontology*. It further tells us always to think about the way how we do our research – *methodology*. These philosophers, especially Plato and Aristotle have been the grandfathers – let me say – for the *success* of Western science and also for the *restriction* of Western science. It's just an example for us. We ourselves also have to think about the ontology of TCM and the methodology that is necessary.

There is another aspect that is different from China: In the Western world Christianity has a big influence to the concept of science and the concept of world. It is the idea that the world is *guided by laws*. Why should there be laws? Chinese people would say that laws are things between human beings. But this is an idea that is coming from Christianity. Even Physicists – like Sir Isaac Newton – have been influenced by Christian thoughts.

1.4.2. Cultural conditions of Chinese science

What is the relation of subject and object in TCM? – This relation is a *way of unification*. You transform the problem of the patient to your own problem. In this situation the Westerner instead refers to his theories, he explains the diseases by applying his theories. Therefore Chinese medicine has a character of *action and construction*. The Western medicine, the strict Western medicine is *applying theories* (a good doctor always does something else beside this too). Therefore we have to be aware that for Western medicine an *additional* ethical reasoning is always necessary. It is necessary that the Western doctor refers to ethics. The Western doctor does not refer to the patient directly; he is referring to a theory. Therefore he has to be aware what is good fort he patient – this is ethical reasoning. In Chinese medicine the ethical reasoning is not necessary because the work of the doctor is *already* ethical.

Now we come to a very important point of the differences between the Western medicine and TCM: The *methodology of TCM is the reasoning of Qu Xiang Bi Lei*. This means that Chinese medicine always is based on the phenomena, on the visual and the imaginable aspects, while the Western medicine always is guided by theories. Chinese medicine is a medicine which uses the *phenomenological aspects of the human being* – one point. The other point is, Chinese medicine is *circular*, it is *not directly* or *linear* as the Western medicine. We have to do a very intensive research in this field.

I am really happy to have somebody here who is researching for instance on fire. What is fire in Chinese medicine? You have to be aware that, if you for instance research Chinese herbs by the ways of Western pharmacology, there are no phenomena anymore. In this way you also get results because the secret of Western methodology is that you always get results. The results may be stupid or wrong but in every way you have results. I want to give you a metaphorical comparison: If you do pharmacology on Chinese herbal systems, you can be compared to someone who analyses the paintings of famous painters by the ways of chemistry of colours. It's nice, but you don't get the result you want to get.

You can see another point: *Chinese language* is a very rich and a very informative system for a culture. Therefore our study has to go back to the Chinese language. I think Chinese language opens a lot of *additional information* – and not only the *language* also the *characters*. Therefore I encourage you – in the case you should do this research in the explained way (I would be happy to supervise it) – go back to a type of *linguistic analysis* of Chinese language.

Here I also would like to refer to the example of chrono-acupuncture which is a good example. It means – as you know – to refer acupuncture to the position of the stars. This is a good example for Chinese holism. For the Westerner it is nonsense, it sounds crazy to him to refer a disease to the position of the star. But it is a good example for holism and for holistic thinking in the Chinese way. We also have to do a lot of research in this field because everybody speaks about holism but this is just a formula. Holism is a *very difficult and interesting way of systematically thinking*.

1.5. Summary

Let us overview this lecture at the end. We had 3 chapters:

1. *What can we expect from science?* – This chapter was an overview of something, a message that is guided by presupposed structures.
2. *The framework of comparison*: The framework of comparison is the position of Constructive Realism. A new, a twenty year old concept in the field of philosophy of science. Compared to the two thousand years history of Europe it is quite new. A new theory of philosophy of science which covers the presuppositions of Western medicine and of TCM.
3. *Cultural conditions of science*: Be aware that experience in the Chinese way is different from experience in the Western way. Therefore you cannot compare the results of a Western research in medicine and a TCM-research directly. We have to find ways of TCM-research which are connected to the original theory of TCM. Otherwise TCM will not be able to survive or could be modernized at least. Therefore evidence-based medicine is a good way to check medical knowledge *in the Western sense* but you *cannot* take the methodology of evidence-based medicine to check the Chinese medicine. For instance: In the Beijing University for Chinese medicine and Pharmacology we have a unit for evidence-based medicine. We must be aware that this is also an important topic for our research. *The direct comparison is misleading*. If you take the evidence-based medicine from the Western research to the TCM, you are going to destroy TCM.

2. Fritz Wallner: Advantages of TCM

2nd lecture at the China Academy of Chinese Medical Sciences in Beijing
14th September 2007

2.1. Introduction

This lecture is very important. It focuses on arguments that we can name to argue our use of traditional Chinese medicine. We're going to go a little bit deeper compared to the last lecture. There are at least five important advantages of TCM, at least five – maybe you find a sixth one. The point of this lecture is: there are *some small similarities to outsiders in the Western thinking*. This is the method we should understand. I bring you together with outsiders of Western thinking which sometimes come closer to the TCM thinking.

2.2. Immediate Experience

The experience of TCM is *without conceptive procedure*. Experience without conceptive procedure means that in TCM *you don't abstract*, you don't go away from the phenomena – *you just take the phenomena as they are*. Compared to this procedure the Western thinking is *always abstracting*; it takes out a few qualities from the phenomena, makes a concept and by this concept it explains nature. This is a way which is *indirect*. – The TCM-way is a *direct* way. I will show you in this lecture a little bit later what is lost if you get used to the Western manner, the indirect way of experience. The TCM-doctor does not leave the phenomena. He remains in the life-world.

A little bit more than hundred years ago there was a philosopher in Europe, original Austrian, later he became German: *Edmund Husserl*. In his works Husserl states what traditional Chinese medicine is always already doing: *Go back to the thing, go to the things directly*. Why did Husserl recommend going back to the things? – Because he recognized that European science was running towards a crisis. One of his famous lectures was titled: „The crisis of European science". I don't want to concentrate on Husserl any further. I just wanted to tell you about Husserl in order to see that the European way is a way which is sometimes leading to a dilemma, to a disaster. Indeed European science had its disaster after Husserl in the seventies and the eighties.

What do we have to conclude from this fact?

1. We have to conclude that it is wrong to look for the way of thinking of Western sciences, if you want to understand TCM.

2. The immediate experience is a treasure which the modern Chinese people have to learn to be aware of. We have to learn to think in this way with the help of the texts. A lot of training is necessary for this request. The training has further to be passed to the students. It will be a lot of training to think in this phenomenological way. It is not easy. Neither for you, nor for us.
3. There is an additional point: TCM has a lot of experience, but this experience has a *different structure* as experience of the Western medicine. Therefore it was a terrible mistake to forget this treasure of experience of TCM or to check this treasure of experience by methods of Western medicine – it would be similar, if we threw our money out of the window. I declare it as the duty of my cooperation with you in the next years to train your methodological thinking. Therefore I also want to give recommendations for a correct methodological thinking in TCM. Methodological thinking in TCM is – as we have seen in the last lecture – *different* from methodological thinking in Western science.

In this lecture I want to give you methodological recommendations: *Don't follow the trivial understanding of TCM as you can find it in many books* – in Western books as well as in modern Chinese books. The trivial thinking about TCM is to say it was just holistic. *This is not wrong, but it is trivial.* Because holism is a habit and if we want to understand TCM or if you want to become real TCM-doctors we also have to learn this habit. You must learn the habit of holism. I am going to tell you different aspects of this habit in this lecture.

Here we also can see one aspect of holism: *Holism is identity between subject and object*. This is just one aspect. This is not just holism. Therefore you may understand that it is nonsense to say: "Let us think holistic. Today we don't think holistic. Tomorrow, next hour we will think holistic". This is nonsense. It is a lot of work to learn the habit, the way of holistic thinking.

2.3. No Reduction of complexity

Maybe you know that in the Western world, in the Western science or also in the Chinese science of today *complexity* is a main topic. Western science is successful because it *reduces complexity*. It makes complex situations easier. Therefore Western science has a quick result, a quick success but it loses a lot by this way. As a consequence of reducing complexity Western science has to deal with side effects. Side-effects are a consequence if you see a complex body situation only in a reduced way. It is an important advantage of TCM that it avoids more side effects by picturing the disease. Therefore you could say: the better a TCM-doctor, the fewer side effects. Sometimes there are also side effects in TCM but this maybe depends on the ability of the doctor. In the Western medicine side effects are *unavoidable*.

I want to illustrate this: The way of *Western medicine*, the theorizing way of Western medicine: You have a lot of examples of symptoms. For example the medical patient has pain. He has different deficiencies. He has problems. He goes to the doctor. What does the Western doctor have to do? He *will not concentrate* on the phenomena the patient offers. Theorize the symptoms! He shall form a theory based on the symptoms. As the next step, the theory has a reduced number of qualities, a reduced number of symbols. The theory is purer than reality in the Western way. The theory has less complexity and therefore less information than the reality. There is *no identity of the elements of the theory and the symptoms – identity is lost*. Therefore thousand or many thousands of patients can be treated by this way and not just one. It is always the same. The Western doctor *deduces* the treatment from the theory. The treatment is a deduction from the theory to the patient.

Let us further consider the situation of the *patient in TCM*. Here you have the same situation. You have a patient with pains, with deficiencies, with problems. He goes to the TCM-doctor. What does he do? He *connects* the phenomena. He does not shift the phenomena to a theoretical level. He connects what he can see, smell and so on. You can see that the phenomena *are not reduced*, the phenomena are still here. Therefore this way is a *more complicated way*, a *slower way*. When he names the treatment based on his diagnosis, he makes a *way of intervention* which we could describe metaphorically as *a new connection between the phenomena*. He finds a new connection between the phenomena. These are the ideas of a genius: to find a new connection between the phenomena to heal a disease. – Here we also have an aspect of holism: *holism as an activity*.

The difference to the Western medicine: We can take a famous formulation of Hippocrates. Hippocrates asks the medical doctor to offer more help than damage. This is Western thinking. The Westerner changes the situation of the body. Therefore he must be aware that he can also damage.

2.4. Considering the historicity of the patient: life world vs. laboratory

What is "historicity"? It names the history, the history of mankind, the history of China. The historicity of somebody is *his own story*, his *own private story*. We all have a story of our life. This is a big difference also to the Western thinking. In the Western world they became aware in the middle of the last century that science should also look to the historical development of knowledge of mankind; and not to believe that only the current position, the present situation is the situation of truth. The ideas of the past were considered as wrong ideas. From this aspect of TCM we can conclude the consequence that *everyone has to be treated differently although they can have similar or the same symptoms*.

Again, be aware about the trivial arguments in the books! The trivial argument is: TCM is better because the doctor has more time for the patient than the Western doctor. This is right, but it is trivial. The real point is that the TCM-doctor has to take the life of the patient and its history into account. Therefore he treats the patient in a different way as the Western doctors that say that they are not interested in the story of his life.

Here you can find an additional important aspect of the holism: *Holism in the concept of the flow of time*. The flow of time is also holistic. It means that the *past is always present* and this is more convenient for the body than just to check the current situation of the body and not to think about all that happened in the last weeks, months or years.

I also want to make a remark about the wrong ideas people in the Western world – as well as in the contemporary China I think – have about TCM. One wrong idea that can be found very often is that TCM is considered as a sample, a mixture of many different medical activities. This is wrong. It sounds right but it is wrong because we can deduce all TCM-efforts from specific principals and from this principal of treatment we can deduce that in TCM we *cannot* divide body diseases from mental diseases.

The division between body diseases and mental diseases is not necessary: I imagine a Westerner who works in the following way: Can we *connect body diseases with mental diseases*? – *Sigmund Freud* is also an outsider of Western thinking. He is not typical for the Western thinking. Freud tried to introduce a bridge between body and mind. He named this bridge "unconsciousness". It is a contradiction in itself. All Westerner said: This is nonsense but this thought was trying to create a bridge from the body to the mind. Therefore Freud did not succeed at the end. He remained unclear because unconsciousness is neither mind, nor body; because the Western world does not offer a system of thinking that can be used for his goal. Therefore these problems are not solved until today. Mental diseases can be treated by the way of *overestimating the body*, by psychopharmacology or they can be treated by the way of *underestimating the body* by speech therapy, by talking with the patient – two different ways. TCM does not have such a division.

In respect to TCM we can speak of an *ontological holism* here – holism in respect to the given world. Here mind is *a part of* the given world. Here we have the fourth meaning of holism – I remind you.

2.5. The intentionality of the patient

Let us go to the next point. This fourth point is the most impressive one to me because here the Western medicine fails – *in the question of human intentionality*. Based on his science the Western doctor only cares about the body of the patient. But we are not only body – more important are our desires, our motivation, our plans, our self-understanding, our self-respect and so on. Why does TCM sometimes look similar to philosophy? People could ask now: Are we in a medical institute or in a philosophical institute? Here you can see one reason why TCM has so much to do with Philosophy. Because thinking about intention is a typical philosophical topic.

The question of human intention is also the argument why we cannot computerize our thought principally. This will be valid for all times. Even in hundred years it will be impossible to computerize thought because intentions are always something which is unexpected by definition. These are the boarders of our artificial intelligence.

Also in the Western philosophy you find a good example for these problems. A very good one is about Socrates written by Plato. Socrates – as you know – was put to prison because he was sentenced to death because they did not like him. Socrates is sitting in the prison and says to his students: "I am not sitting in the prison because my muscles have a specific position. This is not the reason why I am sitting her. The reason is that I want to accept the penalty". – This is *intentionality*.

Probably only a few of us or even nobody of us will come to prison. Therefore I give you an example from our everyday life. A woman comes to the doctor. She has a big problem with her relation to her partner. Therefore all her intentional thinking focuses on questions of this topic: What should I do? What should we do? – This is her real important problem and she maybe has problems with the stomach. The doctor treats the stomach but cannot see and cannot solve the real, the important problem.

2.6. Relativity: Relations are more important than things

The Western thinking focuses on things. Therefore they go to the things, to the element of the things, to the particles, to the electrons and so on. They are always directed to things. As a consequence it was such a big, incredible jump for physics when Einstein claimed to concentrate on relations. Traditional Chinese medicine is always looking for relations at first and then it focuses on things. Therefore we can say the *ontological structure of TCM is relativity*. This is similar to colours. The colours are relations to the light.

These are the five points I have promised. I hope that you got some ideas and gathered some information.

3. Fritz Wallner: The research method in medicine

3rd lecture at the China Academy of Chinese Medical Sciences in Beijing
21st September 2007

This topic is a little bit abstract but you have to know about it and you have to understand it. Otherwise you are going to have problems and biases in your every day practice.

3.1. Principles of our comparison

Every day in China and also in the Western world TCM is compared to Western medicine. But this comparison takes a wrong way very often. Therefore I first would like to explain the principles of such a comparison between these two different systems.
1) *Avoid simplifications*: I give you an example: If the Westerner say that TCM is holistic, this is not wrong. It is a simplification as I already showed you in my last lecture. In this way it is easy to get a comparison that is misleading because in this situation the Westerner usually offers examples based on his understanding of holism that is not adequate to the Chinese view. In this lecture I will offer an example for this statement.
2) *Do not concede the superiority without arguments*: This happens nearly everywhere. In my observations on comparisons of TCM and Western medicine Western medicine is always taken as the normative system, as the system which is without any doubt and based on this system you should check your medicine. This attitude is misleading, this is a mistake. But this mistake is based on the wrong terminology that Western medicine is science and TCM is not science; that it is culture or something else. *But this is nonsense*. Actually as you have seen in my last lectures TCM has a highly elaborated structure. Therefore TCM is *also science – but in another sense, in a different sense compared to the Western medicine*. As a consequence we find the third principle of comparison:
3) *Be aware of your own standards*: I give you an example: The Westerner is not able or not willing to understand „xi jang bi lei". In that case you cannot discuss with him, this is clear. If he says, this is nonsense or this is not scientific, I recommend stopping the discussion.

3.2. The structure of the Western science

Let us first take a look to the structure of the Western science. You have to understand the structure of Western science; you also have to understand the good and the bad aspects, as well as the advantages and the deficiencies of Western science. It's the procedure of Western science *to reduce qualities*. I give an example for the reduction of qualities that is typical for Western science: For instance you have the Newtonian mechanics in physics – I will describe an example that sounds a little bit crazy: If a bad person throws a cat out of the window, then this cat falls according to the laws of Sir Isaac Newton. But in real life this cat will always land on her four feet. The behaviour of living systems is excluded in this type of science – also in the Western medicine. As far Western medicine goes with Western science aspects of living systems are excluded by the way of the thinking of Western science.

The Western science has *three levels*: *First* the level of the *theoretical concepts*, *second* the level of the *empirical data* and *third* the *formal language*. – But I feel obliged to say: if we want to be exact we better should say: theoretical concepts and convictions about science. It depends on the theoretical concept which empirical data can be taken. Empirical data always already depend on the theoretical concept. Therefore you cannot find as a result of your research what is not included in your theory. If you don't have some specific aspects of living systems in the theory, you cannot find this in your result. Please keep this in mind. This is one big deficiency of Western medicine. We always have to be honest and name the advantage of medical systems. In the last lecture I told you about the advantages of TCM but we also should check its deficiency.

In the modern Western science the empirical data are mostly taken by machines – as you know. Here we find a certain problem: Machines are much more detailed, much stricter into tiny particles – but they cannot watch some aspects we see with our ordinary, everyday look. This is another deficiency of Western science, if it is used in Western medicine. Replacing the eyes by the microscope for instance is a *progress* in a way, but it is also a *loss* in another way.

Language is very important for every science as it is used to express the results. In Western science languages are usually formal. I give an example: about ninety years ago there was a big change in one of the Western sciences. It was the change from the so called natural history to biology. Natural history is usually using *every day language*. Biology is already using *formal language*. Therefore people say that a science that is using a formal language is *exact*. A science that does not use a formal language is *not exact*. But as you already know from my former mentions formal languages lose a lot of meaning by the way of abstractions. Therefore they are more useful to get some simplified survey or they are more useful to govern phenomena, to rule phenomena – but they are less useful for understanding. If understanding is an important aspect of living systems formal languages are not so good to describe living systems. Therefore don't be lead astray by the statements of the Westerners that their offer to China medicine is exact. Yes, sometimes or even mostly it is – but it also *reduces a lot of meaning.*

I want to explain that theoretical concepts divide the empirical data and that they already exclude some empirical data as shown in the example of the cats. Some empirical data are not able to be included to specific theoretical concepts. This is the first step. As a second step some empirical data get part of a process of "linguistification". It means that they get a linguistic structure. In the real everyday research both steps are mostly together. Data can be identified by the use formal languages. We can name examples from the field of physics: for instance electrons or atoms.

I also want to explain how success in research is possible. You have to have a heuristic idea for research, at least one. For example: in classical physics the idea, the concept of gravitation can be considered as a heuristic idea. But be aware: nobody knows whether gravitation exists. Gravitation is a concept we just can observe by effects. Therefore you have to be aware that in the Western science the reference to empirical data is always restricted by specific theoretical concepts. The heuristic idea enables the scientists to find a structure for their empirical data. And this structure introduces rules to nature. This is the way of Western science. Rules and laws are invented to explain some phenomena of nature. Always be aware that this is the basis of Western medicine. Also in Western science as well as in Western medicine there is a part which is invented and which is fiction.

A scientific structure can be high levelled as well as it can have the status of low levelled. What is the principle to determine the status of a scientific structure? We can say: *The more the heuristic idea is able to explain, the higher the status of a scientific structure.*

To illustrate this let us think of the concept of gravitation. Based on the idea of gravitation Sir Isaac Newton could explain the movements of earth and the movement of stars. All movements that have a specific structure can be explained with the principles of gravitation. Therefore this principle was a principle of a genius. You have to find just a certain principle that is able to explain so many different things.

In our situation we also can ask: Do we also have such a principle in Western medicine? My answer is: no. I will explain it a little bit later. Clearly we have such principles. I will give you some examples later. But we do not have a principle that is able to explain the whole living systems in such a wide way, a principle that is able to describe and explain all phenomena. This is not possible in Western medicine. The point is that living systems have much more complexity as a system of physics or chemistry. Therefore physics and chemistry can only be applied to living systems in *restricted sense.*

The difference between Western medicine and physics is that Western medicine has less ability to explain because the Western medicine is still mainly inductive. In the first lecture I already told you about the concept of "induction". Induction is the way from the single case to the more general description. In physics you can describe a lot of phenomena by the use of formal language. In Western medicine you have to refer to the single cases very often. But be aware: The Western medicine is more likely to *collect* single data than to *explain* them. We can ask now: Why does Western medicine think in way?

It acts in this way because it has the problem that the complexity of living systems cannot be explained with a few principles. Therefore the Western medicine makes the trial of holism by adding data. But be aware that *this is not holism in the sense of the TCM*. Therefore if the Westerner is speaking about holism he means a *different concept*. I remind you to my reflections about Chinese holism in my last lecture[1]. But as you probably see a way of holistic reasoning is necessary for every medical system because otherwise we cannot draft the living systems. But the difference is that the way of holism of the Western medicine is *artificial*, is *more constructive*. The way of holism in TCM is *natural* – it accords to the thinking of this system.

3.3. Scientific structure of TCM

To start with this chapter I want to name an anecdote: Nils Bore, a great physicist, one of the fathers of Quantum theory, invited philosophers of the Viennese university to a conference in Copenhagen, Denmark. But these philosophers were very shy when they saw this wonderful, theoretical and not understandable system of modern physics. Therefore they did not want to say or to criticize anything. They just agreed. In this situation Bore was shocked. He said: if somebody agrees to this absurd looking system without any protest, he does not understand anything. Therefore if you are not upset about the incompatibility of TCM and Western medicine, you did not understand my lecture. You must tell your friend: there are two different worlds – the Western medicine and the TCM.

Phenomena: It is essential for TCM to focus and to refer to the phenomena. In TCM you don't collect data. In TCM you don't divide into different data. Instead in TCM you are *connecting* phenomena. You should understand that this is another world and that it is different from the way of Western medicine.

There are also great heuristic ideas in TCM. One idea is the idea, the concepts, the *system of the meridians*. This would be a wonderful field for young people to research. I want to tell you how. How could the old genius, the old masters of TCM find out the system of meridian2000 years ago? – Surely not in a similar to Western science. This is clear. They did not have some concept at first and af-

---

[1] See "Fritz Wallner: Advantages of TCM", page 35.

terwards they checked the data. And they say: Oh, here is something and here is something. In this way they would have found out the meridian system.
There must have been a total different way. I give you a hint. – I owe this hint to Dr. Zhang Weibo. Therefore he is also responsible and he has the honour to influence my thinking. It is not only my own invention. But I am not sure, if I am right. This is just a recommendation for research. – I think they found the meridians by a way which is similar to the meditation. If you get in a situation where everything unimportant does not bother you, it is possible that you have a sensation of your body that makes the condition visible for such a deep status of being. In other words, it will only remain what cannot be taken away. By this way some of the genius in the history of TCM might have found the idea that there is a system on the surface of the skin, on the surface of the body, which is basic for what happens in the body.

It is clear that this was not the only way to find out the meridians. There were two other conditions. The first condition is the *Chinese holism*. The Chinese holism teaches us that we must not divide the body. Therefore we must concentrate on the whole surface of the body because only the surface is undivided. If you go inside, you already perform a cut. This is one condition for this heuristic idea. The other condition for the effect of this heuristical idea was the *empirical truth*. Clearly as soon as this insight became common, they made some observations or experiments with them. You don't agree? We should discuss this idea. This is one trial of explanation. Maybe historians of TCM know more, and then we should discuss it. But it is an advice for you to do a research on this question. I just want to underline that this is experience. This is not fiction. But it is experience in a different way to the experience in the Western world. Therefore you cannot apply the concept of the Western world to the meridians. Therefore the meridians cannot be compared to the neural system and it is so hard for the Westerner to accept this concept of meridians because we cannot find them in the way of Western research. But on the other hand for everyone who knows acupuncture it is evident that there is a system of meridians. Therefore think about this example! This is another way to research, to modernize the TCM. Clearly we have to use a lot of knowledge here. You also can research the history of medicine, the history of TCM. In this research we also have to apply the theoretical structure of TCM. Therefore if you for instance carry out a research in the way of modern physics on meridians, you make a Strangification. I recommend doing a Strangification. But be aware that you don't explain them in the direct way.

3.4. The question or problem of evidence based medicine

You know that there are a lot of people in the Western world and also some in China who say that evidence based medicine also has to be applied to TCM. I want to answer this question: Does it have to be applied to TCM or not? – But at first I have to explain: Why does Western medicine need the structure of evidence based medicine?

The Western medicine has – as I already told you – inductive structure. Induction requires observation and observation can fail. This is one reason why the Western medicine needs evidence basis – because the single scientist or also a group of scientists always can fail principally. They can make a mistake in their observation or neglect something which is really important.

But for the Western medicine there is even a more important reason to refer to evidence: The Western doctor has to use his own diagnosis and treatment and his own experience which science does not offer. As I have explained before the living systems, especially the human systems have a lot of aspects which cannot be treated, which cannot be discussed by Western science. Therefore the Western doctor has to deal with two respects: on the one hand he has to consider his science, his scientific knowledge, while on the other hand he has to take his practical experience with patients into account. And this practical experience is clearly an individual experience of the doctor and therefore it can be banned from private opinions.

As a consequence evidence based medicine is necessary to avoid that the Western doctor is mislead by private opinions, by private convictions. Again the scientific structure cannot cover the whole field of medical treatment. The medical science cannot offer the bridge from theory to praxis. It cannot fill the gap between the scientific knowledge and the every day problems that occur while treating patients. Therefore it is a good thing for Western medicine to avoid the influence of private convictions in the treatment of human beings.

Let us take care of another important question: Does evidence based medicine guarantee the truth only by statistical probability? – This is a good question. This would be the best situation. If we have an instance which guarantees that the doctor carried out a true diagnosis, that he used the right treatment and so on. The evidence based medicine only offers *statistical probability*. Therefore if a Western doctor is very careful, he must tell the patient for instance: In 60% of the cases your disease will be healed by this treatment, but in 40% not. And the patient himself can decide if he takes this treatment under these conditions. But if he takes this treatment, and he is one among the 40%, then he has bad luck. You see evidence based medicine is also only a pool.

Why can evidence based medicine not be applied to TCM? To answer this question we have to refer to the TCM concept of Qu Xiang Bi Lei. Qu Xiang Bi Lei is always an individual picture the doctor creates of his patient. There is no gap between the theory and the practice. The TCM-doctor is always looking for single cases. Therefore statistics can not be applied. The reason for his success is another one: How good is his knowledge about the possibilities of TCM and how good is his cooperation with the patient in the unification with the problems of the patient? Therefore you can make a ranking between TCM-doctors. Does he apply TCM in an elaborated way or more in a simple way? But here you don't need and you even cannot refer to evidence basis. Evidence is always present in the real TCM-treatment and TCM-diagnosis. Evidence is always present in the real diagnosis in the real treatment of TCM. *Evidence is not a problem for the TCM-doctor.* The problem could only be his deficiency in TCM, in knowledge and praxis.

The observation of a TCM-doctor is a connection between him and the patients. It does not separate single qualities or single manifestations. Therefore the influence of private convictions in this situation is *much more improbable*. In this case the influence must change the whole system of treatment. And this seems more absurd.

I think I have explained two important ideas. The first one: the difference in the scienticity, in the scientific structure of Western medicine or Western research. And second: evidence based medicine cannot be applied to TCM. – If you understood these two ideas of my lecture, you would have good conditions for discussions with Westerners about TCM.

4. Fritz Wallner: How to Establish an Integrative Medicine?

4th lecture at the China Academy of Chinese Medical Sciences in Beijing
28th September 2007

4.1. Introduction

Let us focus on the question: *How is a good cooperation between Western medicine and TCM possible?* It starts with the real situation. The real situation is insufficient. But before we start I name the chapters of this lecture so that you have an idea of the course of our thinking:
1. Alternative practice
2. Problems of addition
3. Ways of proving systems
4. The principle of equivalence
5. Ways of understanding

4.2. Alternative practice

Let us start with the reality in the Western world: A patient goes to the Western doctor at first and if the Western medicine fails, he goes to a TCM-doctor. By this manner TCM gets the outlook of a *supplement* and this is – as you know – *highly underestimating the possibilities of TCM*. This also has the bad aspect that TCM receives a function as psychotherapy had in the Western world in former decades. Here you can learn about a typical style of Western thinking: First go to the science. If science fails, make something like witchcraft or esoteric or TCM. This is very bad because in this case the practice of TCM gets near to the irrationality or even to witchcraft. But you have to understand: This dichotomy is Western style of thinking.

If you build up on this dichotomy, you will underestimate your own system. This is not a way of a good partnership. This is the way of governing the other one. The praxis of quality assurance is based on this understanding. (I will concentrate on this a little bit later.) The Westerners ask for quality assurance because they want to say TCM is something doubtful.

Intuition is principally a good thing. But if all is based on intuition, it is problematic because there are some doctors who are not gifted with intuition. I know for instance a doctor from Germany for orthopaedics. He has ideas about TCM-combinations. I could not determine and nobody could determine directly, if his combinations are wrong or right, when he for instance relates some diseases of women's back. But this is one striking example why intuition is insufficient. We must find reasonable ways what is possible in the framework of TCM and what is impossible.

The doctor has to have reasons for recommending a specific TCM-therapy instead of a specific Western therapy. But if these systems are incommensurable, a direct way of recommendation is not possible. Just to say: "if one fails, try the other one" – this is too less. Beside TCM we also have Ayurveda or Tibetan medicine – other systems which are incommensurable too. But I don't want to overstrain you. At the end of this lecture you will get a good recommendation how to do it.

4.3. Problems of addition of these both systems

The topic about interferences is more and more discussed in the Western world because a lot of people – about 15%, expressed in numbers this is a huge amount of people – chose both treatments. They sometimes combine acupuncture with Western treatment. But this is a naive way. It would be the same, if someone said: if a medicine is good, I use the double dose. You understand that this is nonsense. More people often use Qigong and Western treatment together because in the Western world you have the wrong idea that Qigong is something like gymnastic. Gymnastic is always good but you can imagine that here can be really big interferences. Therefore one consequence is important for us: *It is necessary to make these interferences part of research*. But to understand these interferences you have to understand the TCM-theory. It is still an insufficient way, if you prove it with Western methods.

4.4. Ways of proving

The Sino-Austrian-Conference that took place here two weeks ago concentrated mainly on *ways of proving*. Let me name and explain different ways of proving:
1. *Internal proving*: For TCM internal proving means to *prove TCM by TCM*. This is a way to have the chance to have much more good aspects than the other ones. But what to do? You have to find a way a TCM-doctor is able to supervise another one. This is a usual way in Western medical systems which are doubtful – for instance in psychotherapy. They do not have ideas of proof as for instance in psychoanalysis and in speech therapies.

   You can imagine how absurd the intention is to prove TCM by Western methods. In the Western world no psychotherapist would agree that his way of psychoanalysis is proved for instance by the way of some mechanisms in psychology. Therefore they have their own way of supervision and another person who is able to handle this practice supervises the doctor. This is one way of quality assurance which is *methodologically correct*. You already have this idea slightly in TCM-practice. According to my experience – which cannot be compared to your experience – TCM-practice is not similar to

Western medical practice in the way that there is just one relation between the doctor and the patient but sometimes – according to my observations – this treatment is opened for the intuitions of the doctor. Different persons are making advices. This is just one way. I do not recommend it, but this is a practice which can lead to supervision.

2. *Quality assurance*: If we speak about quality assurance everybody thinks that this proves TCM with methods of Western medicine and pharmacology. At the conference nobody stands up and says: Why do you do this? What can be the result of such a proof? The result can only be that this therapy does not damage according to the Western medicine. Therefore it nearly says nothing about TCM. By this way you *reduce your own system*. Be aware that all these pharmacologists and people from pharma-firms who are now interested in TCM will lose every interest in you and your system as soon as they have their information; and nothing will be left from the original ideas of TCM. Therefore we should argue in a correct way. In the sense of every methodology this procedure is insufficient. In the Western world nobody would form an own therapy based on that because it mixes incommensurable systems.

To illustrate this in a popular way: You cannot compare apples with pears. This is integration just for the law. In the Western world it has only the sense to protect the doctor against patients that get problems from their treatment. In the Western world this reasoning is always important. If for instance the patient dies after a treatment, it doesn't evoke juridical consequences for the doctor, if he can prove that he fulfilled his work according to the state of science. But nobody discusses if another treatment would have helped. This is an example for reducing medical treatment to a juridical intervention.

3. *Proving vice versa*: This is my message. If you make a quality assurance of your system by Western medicine, Western medicine also has to tolerate a quality assurance by *your system*. This thought leads to the methodology I will explain at the end of this lecture; a methodology that is the key for all these activities. I think that you should take incommensurable systems together – *in a specific way*. But at least it has to be conceded: if you consider one system with the method of the other one, the way of proving vice versa has to be conceded too. But this is not just about fantastical messages. Somebody could think, oh this is so far from reality. But we already did it in the last lectures. I want to remind you to my second lecture[1]. In this lecture I named a lot of examples how Western medicine can be proved by TCM. I showed you the advantages of TCM. This proof is possible and makes sense. But before I explain this methodology in details I would like to teach you these principles that you should consider all the time.

---

[1] See "Fritz Wallner: Advantages of TCM", page 35.

4.5. The principle of equivalence

You have to be aware that there are no convincing reasons for ranking cultures. In the Western world it is common to speak about so called "primitive cultures". This is a terrible nonsense. Even if you travel to so called "primitive culture" for instance in Australia, you can be surprised what they established – for instance in the field of technical aspects, of world views. They also have a highly elaborated language. But it is different from the European world. But this is one of the big mistakes that are surely not going to be corrected in the Western cultural theories. All the time they spoke about development, about high and primitive cultures. This division is very uncertain. There may be some primitive cultures but some cultures that are considered primitive are not primitive at all.

We can learn from this experience that a comparison between cultures has to be done in *another way*. It can not be done in the way of the so called cultural sciences, cultural sciences that apply the Western methodology to describe other cultures. This can only show a very one-sided view. Therefore my suggestion is: *Strangification*. By the way of Strangification we can learn advantages and deficiencies of cultures: For instance by which way a culture can lead to social isolation of people? By which way a culture increases the difference between poor and rich? This difference increased continuously until it was finally spread over the whole world as the Western culture is introduced all over the world. Also in China you can see that these differences become bigger and bigger. This is just an example: What can we learn from cultural Strangification? Another example would be the fact of corruption. Which cultural behaviour leads to corruption? And so on.

Therefore it is a better way to *accept the equivalences of cultures*. Based on this principle we first can *deduce tolerance*. But this is just a method to cover our inability to compare cultures directly. This would mean for TCM: As long as they cannot name deficiencies of TCM they have to tolerate it. Not the other way. As long as we cannot show that TCM is as good as Western medicine we can use it. This principle is very important for your own work. Therefore I use the last part of in this lecture for the most important thought.

4.6. Ways of understanding

First it is clear that full integration of medical systems is an ideal which we cannot reach. But we can come closer to this ideal, if we understand the other systems. Understanding cannot be done by proving the other system by the own system. Understanding mostly means that I agree with you – but this is a reduction of understanding. The understanding of cultural systems – for instance a medical system like TCM – first needs to *refer to life world* because every scientific system *originates from life world*. This is an important thought that even Albert Einstein told us. It is not an outcome of some cultural romanticism. It is also valid for Western science as well as for other sciences. Life world simply *means* our everyday world, the world in which we live in certainty. As life is going well we are living in certainty. We have no big questions. But very often life is not going well. Therefore we need some systems to explain, to help – like medical systems. Therefore we can only understand a system, if we refer it to its founding life world. You also may understand the Western medicine a little better because in the Western world – as I already told you in the former lectures – the reference to the data, to what can be object of physics and chemistry is the most important conviction about the world. What cannot be referred to data is doubtful for the Westerner.

But with TCM the situation is different. TCM refers to a life world which is not present anymore. It refers to a world which does not exist now. Therefore this is one argument that modernization is necessary for TCM. Otherwise we would become what Westerners sometimes suspect us to be that we praise a type of cultural romanticism. I myself made the experience in discussion with colleagues and other people in the Western world several times that they believe that my enthusiasm for TCM is inspired by the enthusiasm of a fantastic old world. But this is wrong. My enthusiasm is inspired by the experience that *totally different world views are possible*. This is an argument how rich the mind of the mankind is. So many different ways are possible – *not just one*.

Now let us go to an essential and difficult question: *What can we do, if we want to understand an incommensurable system?* – For this way I can recommend the method which I developed in philosophy of science about twenty years ago: the methodology *Strangification*. Strangification is a procedure of philosophy of science which takes incommensurable systems together.

Erwin Schrödinger, a famous Physicist from Austria, a winner of the Nobel price was doubtful about the quantum theory. He made a thought experience about the cat which would be dead and alive at the same time according to different observations and according to quantum mechanics. – What can we learn from this experiment? One consequence would be that quantum mechanics is nonsense – but this would be a very primitive consequence. This is the consequence of some Westerners about TCM. We can learn from this experiment that quantum mechanics does not fit into the context of observation in the way of classical mechanics. It does not follow the concept of classical mechanics.

But in this case we have to make the other experiment too and show in which aspect classical mechanics does not follow the quantum mechanics. This is an experiment of applying the principal of equivalence. Only if we apply the principle of equivalence, you can understand this experiment fully.

I tell you about a very personal experience that should show you the application of this experiment to TCM. It was 1993 when I was in Taiwan and at this time I got problems with my back and went to the TCM-doctor to acupuncture. The problem was solved very soon. But the doctor told me that he wanted to check my health totally in the way of TCM. The result was terrible for me because it said that my health was in great danger. I was requested to make a treatment immediately! But I had to return to Vienna to do my duties at my University. Therefore in Vienna I went to my doctor, to internal medicine and asked him: "Please make all the checks you can make and look what is happening in my body!" And he could not find anything. Therefore at this point people usually think: Okay, the TCM-diagnosis was wrong. But as you know TCM-diagnosis does not check the body in the Western sense, but all what is connected for instance to intentionality. Although for Western medicine my body was healthy at this time, my situation was a very bad one. My wife had cancer in the last state and we looked around what can we do? We did not know and I also was in the situation that I have to decide which treatment is right now? What can we do? I believed that this TCM-doctor made a good diagnosis. – This is Strangification. He made a diagnosis about my situation and not just about the functioning of my body.

Now I tell you some more details about Strangification: For the next research it is the best way to make different plans for specific Strangifications. I give you an example: *We take one system into the context of the other one.* For instance you can carry out a Strangification about *Pi in TCM* and *spleen in Western medicine*. Then you can see how both systems are function in a different way. This is just one example. With this example I made a personal experience with a famous Professor of University of medicine in Vienna. My doctor and friend in TCM Mrs. Kubiena told him about Pi and he proved all this by his Western methodology. Some days later he told us at the end: "This is nonsense". His mistake was that he did not use Strangification. He just used quality assurance.

In this way you have a lot of different examples especially for instance in herbal theory. For instance you can take one herb which is used for important treatments and show which connections, which functions this herb has in this treatment. Then take it into the context of Western medicine. Then you will see that they take out just one component. I think that even people who doubt TCM can be convinced by this way that this methodology of approving is nonsense. For example you will not understand a famous Philosopher like Emanuel Kant, if you just count the letters in his book. In this field a lot of research is possible, adequate research is possible and I think this research is necessary for the survival of TCM. In many TCM-institutions I saw that some of the researchers mix the Western methods with methods of TCM. – Strangification is important because by this way you can see the *implicit presuppositions of the system* which is *silently presupposed without any discussion.*

5. FRITZ WALLNER: MODERNIZATION OF TCM WITHOUT WESTERNIZATION

Lecture at the Chinese Academy of Chinese Medical Science
7th March 2008

Thank you for the nice welcome. I always feel happy to be here. Today I have the duty to show you our newest results about the foundations of TCM. Prof. Chang Weibo from your academy participated in this research work of the last months. What I am telling you today is nowhere published until now.

5.1. Introduction

I know that the fist part of this title is a provocation for some people because they don't like the term "modernization" at all; because you know better than me that today in China "modernization" is understood in the sense of abusing TCM. But beside our claim to avoid any abuse we have to look for modernization by different reasons. Modernization of TCM does not mean that we want to change the rich body of the tradition of TCM for instance the work of I (Nei) Jing. It would be nonsense and crazy as well to intend to change these ideas. Instead we want *to make TCM fit in three respects*:

1) *The correct application of Western science to TCM*: One aspect which is unavoidable today is the question how to apply Western science to TCM in a correct way. You cannot say we want to be separated from the whole world because all over the world you have Western science. We have to face it with open eyes. Instead TCM has to be supported to play a fair game with the Western science, to use the Western science correctly.
2) The second aspect is *the adequate modernization of TCM*: This means that the contemporary society is different from the society of classical China. This even means – as you know better than me – that teaching of TCM today is usually a university teaching and not the master teaching of the old times. Therefore you have a style of teaching which is adjusted to the Western way of teaching: You also have to adapt the presentation of TCM.
3) This lecture today *offers a paradigm for your cooperation in future*: Prof. Chang Weibo and I formed a type of "scientific couple" in Vienna. We performed a scientific cooperation face to face – this should be done several times for different topics in the future. Later he will present his topic and some of you maybe can be the next one this autumn who cooperates with me and we can present another topic next time.

5.2. The structure of Western science

I do a very short review about the structure of the Western science which is incompatible to the structure of TCM. The core of Western science are the procedure of a) *induction* – it means to go from the single case to the general proposition or general theory – and the one of b) *deduction* – it means to take the other direction, from the general theory to the single case. Therefore the work of a doctor in the Western world is different to the work of TCM-doctors. They have another education which is incompatible to TCM. I want to underline this point: We have to make our students to become aware that if they become doctors, they act in a *different way than the Western doctors* – otherwise they don't perform TCM. For example they can make acupuncture, but this is not TCM what they are doing for instance.

There is a third point: *The difference in the concept of reality*. In English language we even cannot express it completely because they have only the term "reality". If we use the German term "Wirklichkeit" beside "reality", we can name a wonderful, fascinating difference in the concepts of reality. But I will tell you about this later.

5.3. The core structure of TCM

At first let us focus on the methodology of *Qu Xiang Bi Lei*. Qu Xiang Bi Lei is a way of presenting reality which is different from the Western way of presenting reality. In the Western world the image is only a *model*, it is only a tool to get to reality; while in Qu Xiang Bi Lei the image is *essential*. Taking images from nature is as taking out the essence of nature, the essence of objects, not just models of object. Further we do not go to different levels of abstraction. We connect these images to a *circle*. Therefore it is easy for everybody who understands Qu Xiang Bi Lei that contradiction has no importance here or that contradiction has a different function than in the Western thinking. In the Western thinking contradiction means: One is true and the other one contradicts the first so one must be wrong. In Qu Xiang Bi Lei contradiction means that an image becomes more colourful by contradicting one – it means that a contradiction does not lead to an exclusion of the contradicted, instead it opens new ranges of meaning.

A second essential aspect is *the unity of human and nature* (Tian Ren He Yi): In the Western thinking the human being is always in *difference to nature*; man is always *out of nature*. This is the beginning of Western philosophy two thousand years ago that *nature is in contradiction to man*. – TCM thinks both together. For instance take a look at the Chinese gardens all over China: They are a *combination of man and nature*. Man is always present in this garden. Therefore we have to understand here that "reality" or "Wirklichkeit" is a different concept for classical Chinese thinking than for Western thinking. Everyone who studies or who has to apply TCM has to understand at first that the so called "objects", the "reality" are referring to what is given on the one hand ("Wirklichkeit") and that they are constructed on the other hand ("reality) – but *both at the same time*. The images of Qu Qu Xiang Bi Lei are *given by nature and constructed by men*, both together. This different concept of reality is connected to one of the big advantages of TCM in comparison to Western medicine[1]. I already showed you a number of advantages in September. One of them is that with TCM you also take intentions, wishes or fears into account – something that is completely neglected in the Western medicine. In TCM human being is not an *object*, but *in movement*.

5.4. A new philosophy of science: "Constructive Realism"

I want to start to talk about the crisis of modern science and the position of Constructive Realism. I want to name some reasons why this new philosophy of science is so helpful for understanding and for constructing a bridge between Eastern and Western thinking. The position is titled: "Constructive Realism".
Constructive Realism replaces *description* by *construction*. At first our thoughts were based on old ideas by Demokrit that the images are coming from the world. This is an important outcome of modern Philosophy. By this way you can understand both Western science and TCM. I will show you some examples. The Western science has come to a crisis, if it takes the claim of knowledge seriously. You might know that the general relativity theory is teaching us that if the velocity is coming close to the speed of the light, the length of things is increasing and time is reducing. Now we have to ask a question: If I fly with speed of light, do things really get so long or is it just an effect (medical people would call it a placebo of medicaments, an effect of medicaments)? In the Western world no one is able to answer this question because we have an ontology which restricts this answering. I want to underline this because if somebody says: "we have science and you the 'old fashioned' TCM", you can say: "the 'old fashioned' TCM has already known things which they don't understand currently in the Western world".
Another example is for instance the famous and important questions of Western cosmology about the *borders of the universe*. Because nobody can say what is behind the borders – you might know the famous book about the first five seconds of the Universe. This is a typical outcome of Western ontology because what does it mean? What has been before the universe? I name these examples just to give you arguments against people who are narrow-minded and who say: "We have science and other things are fact of believing or fact of everyday knowledge". This is nonsense: We have *two sciences* – first the Western medicine and second the TCM. These are very simple arguments for the *principle of*

---

[1] See "Fritz Wallner: Advantages of TCM", page 35.

equivalence, the equivalence between different cultures, the equivalence of scientific value between Western science and Chinese science.

Let us ask an essential question: Why is it important to take the concept of Constructive Realism into consideration? Constructive Realism can be considered as a bridge between Confucianism and Western thinking: It offers ways to explain each of them.

For Constructive Realism the ontological concept is essential: I already explained it in my lectures in September[2] therefore I don't want to repeat it here. I only want to add a wonderful example which my friend Dr. Wu introduced: *the given world and the constructive world cannot be divided clearly – they are like Yin and Yang*. And this is valid for both Western science and Chinese science. Therefore if we say we have different incommensurable sciences we should not be frustrated. There are bridges possible. But these bridges have to be done by very clever thinking.

What is the difference between Western healing and TCM-healing? There are *different types of healing*. The Western healing is *applying theories to specific cases*. Therefore if one Western doctor says: This is this disease. While another Western doctor says: This is another disease. Then one of them has to be wrong. If one TCM-doctor has made his diagnosis and another doctor has another diagnosis, it can be that one of them is wrong, but it is not sure that one of these diagnoses is wrong – because TCM is a way of *interactive healing*. Therefore every diagnosis is a diagnosis in respect to the healer. You see that here is a problem for teaching TCM. You have to make precautions that the methodology is *applied correctly*. This is a topic for the next October. In the case of TCM I recommend a *type of supervision*. You cannot refuse the other diagnosis by facts – this is the Western way. In the way of TCM you can make clear by supervision if the reflection of the body of methodology is not used correctly. I just wanted to name this because it shows that *different ways of healing are possible*. This is a way of applying TCM to the Western medicine. The idea of TCM of the manifoldness is used here to make the differences in healing understandable.

5.5. Strangification

At first we want to define the term of „Strangification": Strangification means to *take one theory in a total different context*. Therefore the application of Western science to TCM is always Strangification because Western theory is taken to a different context. It is clearly not forbidden to use Western science, but to state that you can explain TCM by Western science is absurd.

---

[2] See "Fritz Wallner: The comparision between Western medicine and TCM", page 27. Also see: "Kurt Greiner, Fritz Wallner: Innovative Ontology and Methodology: An Introduciton into Constructive Realism (CR)", page 17.

If you are aware that the application of Western science is a Strangification for TCM, you can get some interesting results. I already showed you one interesting result in September that TCM takes the intentions of the patient into account. I want to underline this because usually the practitioner is not aware about this. TCM-healing always takes the past and the future of the patient into account – *because of its structure.*

It is a famous mistake in the Western world that they believed (or some of them believe it right now) that meridians are conceptual forerunners for the neural system. But this is wrong and I contend that in no future we are going to be able find something like meridians under the skin by the use of microscopes. Meridians show us that the observer is always included into the process. Otherwise the TCM-healer always has to be afraid that for instance in acupuncture he makes a small mistake, if he puts the needle just one nanometre beside the systematic point – but this is not the sense of acupuncture. I want to remind you that this idea – that the observer is included into the process – is an idea coming from system theory.

5.6. Strangification of TCM by Western science – examples

Prof. Chang had the great idea to introduce the concept of "constructive imaging reality" to underline that Constructive Realism applied to TCM has a different meaning as Constructive Realism applied to Western science. I would like to remain here a little bit because this is very important for the research in the future.

The way from the given world to the constructive world is really different in the Western science than in TCM. In the Western science you come to elements by analysis and local observation. In TCM you come to images and holistic observation by this constructive imaging job. This means to put images in the circle. I just want to underline a typical superficial misunderstanding in the Western world. If you don't have the metodology you cannot come to holism. You cannot come to holism by free will. You have to have a methodology and one methodology is for instance Qu Xiang Bi Lei.

III. Extension: Contribution of other TCM scientists

1. ZHANG WEIBO: STRANGIFICATION OF TCM BY WESTERN SCIENCE: UNDER WHICH CONDITIONS CAN WESTERN SCIENCE BE USED IN TCM CORRECTLY?

Zhang Weibo, Institute of Acupuncture and Moxibustion,
China academy of Chinese Medical Science

1.1. Preface

Nowadays, global economy and internet makes the world smaller and smaller. Different cultures have more chance to dialogue and collide. Medicine with its important role in human health is meeting the challenge of such collisions. Western medicine and traditional Chinese medicine (TCM) are two kinds of medicines which developed many years respectively. How to look at TCM when modernization comes to China? What's going on when TCM spreads to the Western world? Some people think TCM is not a science by the standard of Western science. A big discussion was then induced in China recently. In Europe on the other hand, some criticizers are reconsidering the Western science and Western medicine particularly on a philosophical level. Constructive realism is a now developed science of philosophy originated in Wittgenstein and mainly created by Fritz Wallner from Vienna University during the 1990's. His new view about science and new philosophic methodology of constructive realism has enlightened the development of TCM. Here we discuss TCM by the view of constructive realism.

1.2. What is Science?

1.2.1. Classic Definition of Science

Science has multiple meanings: one indicates the knowledge which is "truth" or "scientific". We called it "scientific knowledge" (SK). The other illustrates an activity which aims at getting SK or a person who is trying to get SK. Another usage for science is in the description of a method as a scientific method by which SK can be obtained.

As the implicit meaning of science in the second and third aspect, we mainly discuss the first one, what is scientific knowledge. In general, SK includes a series of paradigms which descript the structure of world, laws, rules and relations. One function of SK is to explain the phenomena we meet everyday so as to understand the reason of the phenomena. We sometimes refer to the reason as mechanism of the phenomenon. This is the function of SK of "why". The second function of SK is to control the world through a right behaviour or a right technique guided by SK and get predict results. We refer to this function as "how" or "know how".

This definition of science seems to work well until science develops to a very deep layer of micro level. In quantum theory, the location and speed of a presumed electron can't be determined simultaneously. So the pattern of SK in this level is implicit. The position of an electron outside the nuclei can only be described by possibility which is unsatisfying for classic physicians. The other difficulty is the dynamics of multiple body interaction. The equations to describe the movements usually have more than three variables and high rank. The solution may become unstable with chaos status which is sensitive to a very tiny fluctuation in preliminary conditions. It is hard to foretell the behaviour of the system in such a situation.

In medicine, the function of medical knowledge instructs a doctor to deal with a patient as a machine. The cause of a disease is usually simple and direct like the situation in a lifeless world. The treatment is usually towards the simple and direct cause which is adjusted by chemicals or by an operation. This function of "know how" in Western medicine doesn't work well like the prediction in many diseases particularly in chronic diseases.

1.2.2. Constructive Realism

The new proceedings in physics and other disciplines made philosophers think about science again. The Vienna circle in 20th century engaged in building up a logic guarantee to science – but failed. They had to admit that the foundation of modern science has a problem. Wittgenstein who is partly the member of Vienna circle had a logion that the language I use is my world which means that science depends on the language it uses and no one can guarantee that one language is superior to the other. To do a scientific research a presupposition has to be made before the study which is regarded as to be right without verification. The presupposition is also called the prior experience in Kant's theory.

As the description of the world depends on the language and presuppositions which are not reliable by any methods, a new philosophy called "Constructive Realism" (CR) born in Vienna in 1990 which tried to change the idea of describing the world in SK into constructing the world. CR thinks science can't describe a given (real) world. The usual work scientists do is to simplify the world to a few qualities and reconstruct them as a micro-world. The micro-world is not a real world but it can somehow work and can be applied in everyday life. Actually the world is very complex, a separation has to be done to deal with the world and to get knowledge. For example, we have to divide the material into molecule level and atom level. When molecules change, a chemical process was reached while any change inside the nuclei of the atom was ignored. The discipline of chemistry was formed to deal with the laws in this level while inside the nuclei, the laws belong to the physics, particularly atom physics. The whole micro-worlds were thought by CR as the real world but we haven't known how to integrate them, how to put these micro-worlds together yet.

CR suggested a new method called "Strangification". One can put one science (theory, concepts, and paradigms) to the frame of other sciences or different contexts to make the science and the language the science uses understandable. The strangification will benefit both sciences. Such study is also called "interdisciplinary" or "intercultural" in a bigger scale.

1.3. Is TCM a science or not?

By the standard of science mentioned above, science must have the ability to explain phenomena, i.e. to give a reason or argument to the phenomena. This was just what TCM did. TCM theory specifically deals with the reason of disease and health, namely why a disease appears or why some people can live healthy and longer. For a typical example, TCM explains the reason why old people do not sleep well. The reason was that the muscles of old people become unsmooth, the Wei Qi flows without regular speed and circulation. As Wei Qi controls the sleep and awakening while it circulates in Yang channels and Yin channels, the disorder of its circulation causes the old man not to sleep well and to awake without spirit.

By this example, you can see TCM has a very good logic structure to explain physiological phenomena. People in the Western world may argue that this explanation hasn't been verified by Western science. So it is not legitimate. This is totally wrong. Western science tests their legitimacy of science by a system of propositions and logic which has been proven impossible by philosophy of science in the twenties or thirties in 20th century. The other important reason is that we don't know what ancient people meant about the Qi and the channels. So no one can confirm that he has already found a way to prove it doesn't exist, or it is nonsense. Therefore TCM has a characteristic of science.

The second characteristic of science is that it sometimes can be functional, can guide application and predict results. This is just the advantage of TCM which mainly serves as the instruction how to treat diseases. In the history of TCM, a great doctor usually reads thoroughly the classic of TCM and is guided by the classic deeply in treating a patient. TCM provides diagnosis of diseases, the analysis of the cause and the principle of treatment. If you obtain accurate information, the symptoms, and analysis correctly and give a good treatment, the result is usually efficient. If there is an insufficient effect, it is usually not the sake of TCM theory but the process of application of TCM. It is also to consider that not all the diseases can be healed by both TCM and Western medicine.

Like Western science, TCM has also a presupposition system. This system concludes two main aspects. One is called: man and nature are coincident or man follows the nature. This idea comes from long time observing the relationship between man and nature. As man born from nature, ancient people thought man must have a similar structure and similar rules as nature. The idea is not the result of deduction but a transcendental knowledge. Comparing with the irrational presupposition in Western science, this presupposition is more reasonable. The other is Qu Xiang Bi Lei which means similar phases (structure or phenomena) have similar functions which should be grouped the same. This is also a prior experience by ancient Chinese just like the absolute time and space presupposed in Newton's mechanics. The presuppositions support a series of consequences in TCM theory.

So TCM theory has totally scientific characteristics. The reason why Western world don't want to receive TCM as a science is that its concepts are hard to be understood, hard to be coincident with the Western concepts and therefore can't be verified by scientific experiments and examined by Western scientific standard. It is worse for them to think this scientific standard is universal. So the so called "Modernization of TCM" is using Western scientific standard to examine TCM to see if it is correct or not. As the concepts in TCM are mostly not clarified by Western scientists, also by many Chinese scientists, the verification or the study usually fails to predict results and upsets the Chinese while sometimes it is cheerful by Western scientists as they think TCM is impossible to be wiser than Western science and could not provide knowledge which Western science doesn't know. This is a serious prejudice.

1.4. What kind of science is TCM? Comparison with Western medicine

We have argued that TCM is a science. It has all the characteristics of science. But why some people still think it is not a science? The true reason is that TCM is a kind of science which is very different from Western science. The differences are as follows:

1.4.1. TCM gets experiences through man's consciousness comparing with the instruments in Western science

Different from Western science that usually handles a phenomenon by measuring something with an instrument and analyses the data by math, TCM does experiments on the doctor's body and the patient's body. When doing an experiment on the doctor's own body, he will use his own feeling to detect the rule of the disease changed with herbs or acupuncture. We all know the story of testing hundreds of herbs by Shen Nong well. When doing experiments on the patient's body, the doctor detects the changes by asking the feeling from the patient and testing the pulses, the colour of tongue etc. By these two processes, ancient doctors summarized the rules of disease and developed therapeutic techniques.

Western people usually think this kind of study is not objective. But according to CR, Western science is impossible to objectively describe the given world as they choose their presuppositions subjectively and further choose an instrument which is only adapted to watch what they want to watch. Although man's feeling is not as accurate as a machine, it is more objective than a machine because man's feeling detect a holistic situation in human body while an instrument can only access one or two aspects to be observed.

1.4.2. TCM constructs the world by imaging the reality

Also different from Western science, TCM doesn't describe the world by saying what the structure of a disease is or what Qi is. It is usually said, what a disease looks like, where it comes from and where it goes to. For a sick pulse, for instance usually saying, it is similar to hold a pipe of onion etc. The most basic pattern of the world in TCM is Yin and Yang. Yin-Yang and their relations form the world, representing the basic mechanism of the world. This type of world is mostly different from the constructed world by Western science. We could not say which one is better. Both can work on human body to solve a certain extent of diseases. But if one asks which is closer to the nature, I would answer the theory of TCM is closer to the nature, to the reality of diseases.

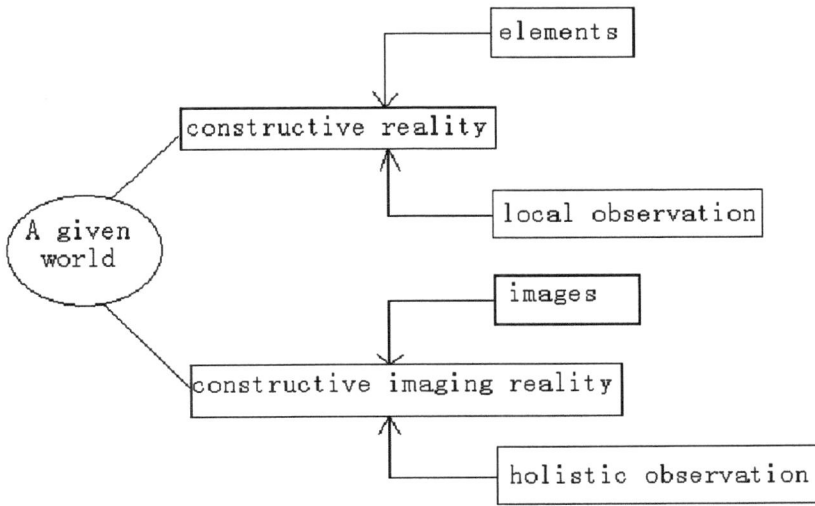

Fig. 1: The relation between constructive reality and constructive imaging reality

There are several approaches to get the pattern in medicine according to the different cultures. Buddhism created a kind of medicine developed in Tibet while Arabian medicine developed in Chinese Muslim called "HuiHui" medicine. All these kinds of medicines construct the medical world in different ways. TCM is a kind of construction. As TCM usually construct the medical world by imaging patterns, we would like to refer to this kind of construction as constructive imaging reality (CIR).

Both CR and CIR construct the given world. The difference is that CR constructs the world by elements while CIR constructs the world by images. The relation can be shown in Fig. 1.

The word "image" (*Xiang*) is a rich Chinese concept which means functional, presenting, phenomenon, information and symbol. A deep study should be made for the Chinese term "image". The imaging reality is a very important methodology in TCM. The use of "imaging" as a verb doesn't mean TCM just imagines reality by mind, by thinking of medical laws randomly. Similar to Western science, TCM observes the nature, body and diseases very carefully and many phenomena or rules (repeatable phenomena) were found. The difference is the way of observation I mentioned above. Apart from self and holistic, the observation usually takes a longer time than Western medicine. A doctor often repeats his experiences on his own body and on patients many many times until he dies and the experience can pass on to his apprentice. Here the apprentice is different from the student in the West. An apprentice must get his master's experiences by heart and by feeling. So the transportation is very difficult and usually between one master and just one or several apprentices. This kind of experience is necessary to get a holistic view of the nature or the diseases while Western medicine can only get part of the nature by local and short observation.

Apart from the holistic observation, TCM images our body under the background of nature which is called man and nature are coincident or man follows the nature. I prefer the later translation as this sentence show the second position of human in respect to nature. This ideology in TCM has the similar function of presupposition in Western science. Although summarized from thousands times of observation between nature and human body, it mainly comes from the believing of the power of nature. Unlike the religion in the Western world that God created everything, ancient Chinese believe that nature created everything including man which is more close to the conclusion of natural science. By modelling the nature, many compounds in human body were named after the compounds of nature. For example, the sweat of Yang in our body was named by rain in nature, the Qi of Yang was named by strong wind in nature. These names are not just the names. They show the similar properties with that of nature. So in Yellow Emperor's Canon of Internal medicine, the author pointed out if we don't follow the laws in nature to treat our body, the disaster will come.

The nature was even used to explain the physiological phenomena in our body. For example, when Yellow Emperor ask QiBo the master of Yellow Emperor why the right ear and eye are not as cleaver as left ones while left hand and foot are not as functional as right ones. QiBo answered that east belong to Yang which goes up, making left ear and eye more cleaver while hand and foot at the same side are less functional. In this explanation, the person must stand towards south, and then his left is in the east side. The interpretation is somehow logical but hard to be proven as we don't know what Yang (Qi) is. It is an imaging concept formulating the nature. TCM provides many imaging concepts and interpretations to the phenomena in our body according to the principle of nature. By the standard of CR, TCM provides knowledge.

1.5. Does TCM need to be improved or not?

TCM has maintained its status and developed slowly for more than two thousands years. The core of TCM has never changed since Neijing. All the developments concerned on how to apply the theory in clinic. The situation implies that the theory is stable and functional. But just in these several hundred years whenever the Western medicine was introduced into China, people began to doubt TCM from its truth even it is still effectively used in society. This procedure has taken for a long time since Japan, the Government of Guomintang and then the People's Republic of China.

One of the reasons in this doubt is that Western medicine provides a different explanation of the diseases which seems clearer and more reliable than TCM. There were anatomic evidences and others from physiological and pathological certifications. The high-tech diagnosis by expensive machine makes people more believe the Western medicine than the diagnosis carried by man in TCM. This influence by Western medicine is also related to the industry. In everyday life, rich products and technology from Western world prove the effects of Western science and convinced the Eastern people that Western science is the truth of the world. The Western science is becoming a new kind of religion which everybody should believe. If you argued with the Western science, you would be thought to be mad. Everybody in the world, even every Chinese now, get education of scientific knowledge throughout their life. Scientific language has become a universal and understandable language which communicates the people in different cultural background.

Nowadays, Western medicine has distributed throughout China and even TCM students learn a lot of Western medicine in college time. Many TCM doctors use Western diagnosis and even Western medicine during the treatments. Experienced TCM doctor are less gradually. People, not only Western but even Chinese doctor don't understand TCM and don't convince TCM. There is a crisis in TCM indeed if there is no change in such a situation. The conclusion is that TCM should be improved or in another word TCM needs an interpretation by

Western science, needs to be better understood and better techniques should be used.

1.6. How to improve TCM rather than negative intervention

1.6.1. The history of improvement of TCM by Western science

During a long time, many people have tried to change TCM since Western medicine and Western science were introduced to China. A famous book, "Zhong Zhong Yi Xue Can Xi Lu" was written by Zhang Xichun in 1920's which is the first attempt to combine TCM with Western medicine. Since 1949, a disciplinary called combination between Chinese and Western medicine has set up as the first level of disciplinary and many scientists work in this field. Some improvements were achieved such as electric acupuncture and new Chinese herbs but until now nobody gets real success to replace the traditional treatment by a new treatment which is totally superior than TCM. Some changes gave a direct writing equal sign between Western concept and Chinese concept, for instance meridians equals to nerve system, which caused a big mistake and wrong guidance to the application that acupuncture can be replaced by transcutaneous electric stimulation. The changes had even negative intervention to TCM such as replacing Chinese herbs by purified Chinese medicine. Such replacement changes Chinese medicine to a kind of Western medicine which was similarly used like Western medicine and has a similar side effect as well. The guideline of this improvement is that Western medicine is superior to Chinese medicine which should be rebuilt by Western medicine. The change of TCM in the idea of Western medicine hasn't improved TCM very much. Conversely TCM became weaker and weaker. So the combination of Western science and TCM must be done very carefully.

1.6.2. Strangification: a new method CR suggests to us

Strangification is a new method created by Fritz Wallner in the 1990ies for better understanding a scientific theory. It is said that to understand a theory, the proposition of the theory should be put into another context of a theory or a science to see what happens. Usually a limitation of the replacement emerges which can give a new and better understanding of the theory. The theory then gets an interpretation.

 A new approach from the author is that if we put the proposition or a concept of a theory into another context of theory or science, several situations may happen. One is that we find it is just a joke, a nonsense that totally doesn't work, that we could not increase our understanding of the theory anymore. Secondly, we find a limitation, in some conditions it is fitted while sometimes it is not fitted or quite unclear. If we want to get it fitted, we must do more works such as to do further experiments to see it is right or wrong. The third situation is that we find that the translation is totally fitted in the new frame of the theory so that we get a very good understanding of the old theory and also the new theory was improved.

1.7. Strangification of TCM by Western science

1.7.1. Two preconditions before a strangification of TCM by Western science

How to put the concepts of TCM into Western science and what will happen after this was done? In 1.4.2 we have pointed out that TCM is a science which is totally different from the Western science. To use Western science on TCM is not easy. Some people think that the concepts used by TCM are just other terms of modern findings it couldn't be two objectives on human body. So they simply change the terms in TCM by the terms in Western medicine. This usually goes to a far more misunderstanding of TCM.

In modern TCM research, the common situation is that people find phenomena in labs which has some relations to the concepts of TCM. And then such phenomena were studied, explained by a mechanism with Western knowledge and then were proved following the guidance of the mechanism. Here the modern phenomena replace the classic concepts of TCM. It is usually thought that scientists can do nothing without the replacement. But the replacement extracts only some parts of the given world, of the real property in our body. A typical example is the concept of meridian. Meridian is a concept where ancient people realized that the human body refers to a channel through which Qi and blood flow. The channel is the imaged production from real or given meridian. For modern people who want to study the meridian, phenomena related to meridian should be studied first. Propagated Sensation along Channel (PSC) is a famous phenomenon related to meridians. But PSC only appears in rare people. Scientists study the PSC by putting forward hypothesis which can explain PSC and prove it experimentally. After the process, a concept of constructive meridian was built to get the idea of meridian. Then it argues that if a person without PSC does it, mean the person hasn't meridian. It is certainly a mistake to construct the meridian instead of the channels in TCM. So the modern TCM phenomena are only the gate of entering TCM. We could say it is a construction to the constructive imaging meridian in TCM. Normally you can find other phenomena related to the meridian and that can be constructed by other constructive realities. The constructive results must be integrated and put back to the frame of TCM to check the fitness with TCM theory. This is the new step we call the integration & interpretation which can make the constructive result more close to the real meaning of imaged meridians in TCM. The process is shown in Fig. 2.

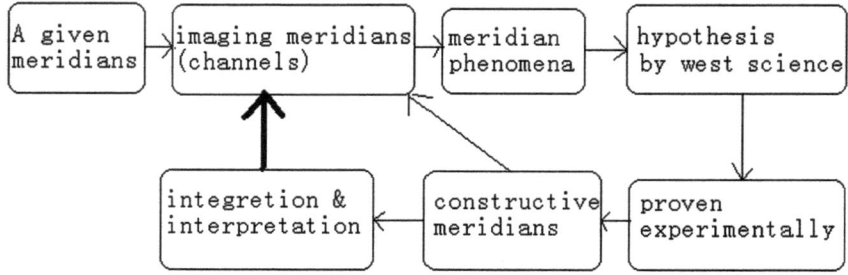

Fig. 2: The process of studying meridians

Finding modern TCM phenomena and studying it with Western science is a way to improve TCM by the guidance of literature study. Literature study is a direct analysis of the The other way is to replace the concepts in TCM by Western science structure of TCM theory, its origin and development. A scholar Huang longxiang in China pointed out that unless we get the experiential fact from the literature, we can put TCM into lab to study. This process was called "getting pears from necklace". This idea is useful when sometimes trying to do experiments. But it ignores the precious thread in a necklace which makes the necklace holistic. The thread also provides the relations with other part of TCM by which we could understand TCM (Fig.3).

Finding modern TCM phenomena and studying it with Western science is a way to improve TCM. The other way is to replace the concepts in TCM by Western science under the guidance of literature study. Literature study is a direct analysis of the structure of TCM theory, its origin and development. A scholar Huang longxiang in China pointed out that unless we get the experiential fact from the literature, we can put TCM into lab to study. This process was called "getting pears from necklace". This idea is useful when sometimes trying to do experiments. But it ignores the precious thread in a necklace which makes the necklace holistic. The thread also provides the relations with other parts of TCM by which we could understand TCM (Fig.3).

Finding experimental phenomena and studying the literature of TCM are both the precondition of strangification of TCM. We can go from one way or from both ways. Usually considering both experimental phenomena and literature experiential fact can reach a good strangification more quickly. Here are two examples of strangification of TCM by Western science.

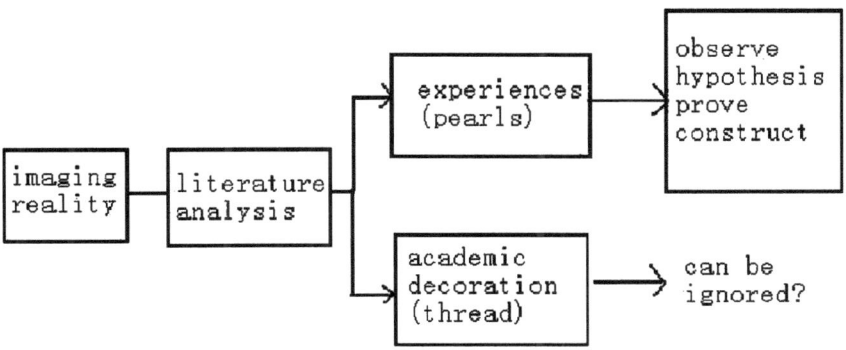

Fig. 3: The literature analysis before strangification

1.7.2. Strangification of meridians and Qi

Some people think meridian is a wrong translation by the first translator. Meridian should be translated to nerve as nerve fibres have a threadlike anatomical structure and parallel position with blood vessels. The Deqi feeling when doing acupuncture is also related to neural impulse. But if we replace meridians by nerve fibres, we lose the meaning of "channel" which is the basic characteristic of meridians. In TCM meridian is the channel in which Qi and blood flow. If we think meridian is a nerve, Qi should be neural impulse. But if we replace the Qi by neural impulse, it loses the basic function of Qi which can moist and nourish the tissue. In TCM Qi originates from our eating and drinking, while it is hard to say neural impulses are produced from our eating and drinking. Also many relations were wrong such as the relations between Qi and blood. In TCM theory Qi can change into blood when Qi goes into the vessel and blood can change into Qi when it goes out of the vessel. The relations between Qi and sweat, urine, tear etc. are not fitted as well. The velocity of Qi is also much slower than neural impulses. So Qi is not simply nerve impulse. But the concept of Deqi is clearly presented that Qi is related to a kind of neural impulse. The conflict induces two consequences. One is that meridian and Qi can't be explained or replaced simply by nerve fibres and neural impulse which is the ontological concepts in Western medicine. The other possibility is that Qi and Deqi are two different concepts, are two kinds of Qi.

In my twenty years study of meridians I tried to replace meridian by interstitial fluid channel. What happened when meridian was replaced by interstitial fluid channel? Firstly I find many relations were fitted like Qi and blood, Qi and sweat, urine, tear and so on. But I also find no similar ontological knowledge in Western medicine, i.e. no anatomic evidence to show such meridian like channel of interstitial fluid exists on human body. During the study of the physiology about interstitial fluid, it was found that the flow of fluid is very unclear and argumentative. So the strangification implies that a new knowledge about interstitial fluid flow may be revealed by TCM. This strangification then became a hypothesis in modern science which can be experimented, having a chance to fail. Fortunately I have proved that there is a low hydraulic resistance channel along meridians and rich interstitial fluid in the channel. The new finding gives a better understanding of the TCM theory in many aspects.

But a new demand arises from Western science in respect to the anatomic structure. Some people ask me to show the structure of the channel. In the fluid channel, the important idea is that the fluid must flow. To fit to the condition of fluid flow, a continuous, long distance low hydraulic resistance and hydromechanic conditions like a converge along the pathway should exist. Although we could find a porous structure in a slice or thousands of slices which could really cause low hydraulic resistance, it could not be said that it was the structure of the channel because of lack of dynamic condition. In the other word, a real fluid channel can only be built by several things as a whole. The limitation of an anatomic view in the Western medicine was found in this strangification. The situation can be simulated by studying the Danube river in Vienna which

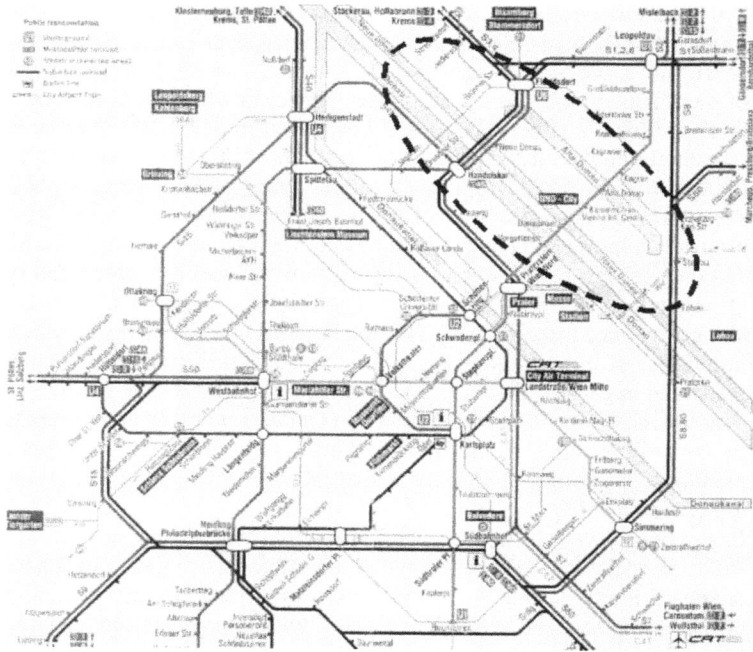

Fig.4: the map with Danube river in Vienna

has several branches (Fig.4). One branch has stases in two sides and became a lake called "Alte Donau". But if we study the structures by intersecting the branches of Danube river, we get the same structures between the real river and the dead river. So the anatomy of river can't explain the property of river. Therefore we understand that meridian or Qi-channel is a functional concept concerning many structures and dynamics. It was imaged correctly by TCM in a way we don't know by now, mostly by self observation of Qi and meridian phenomena on patients. Through this case, we understand that any concept in TCM is complex, functional. It does not come from anatomic observation and can not simply be coincident with the anatomic structure which is the old wrong way we have walked during the forty years meridian research.

1.7.3. Strangification of Yin-Yang and five phases

Different from Meridian and Qi, Yin-Yang and five phases are more abstract concepts in TCM. Many people don't understand what Yin-Yang is. They put Yin-Yang theory into the position of pseudo science in TCM. In the recent years, some scientists tried to translate Yin-Yang and five phases into mathematic concepts, the variables. One of them is my good friend Prof. Yang Xuepeng. He represents Yin-Yang by two variables X and Y, and then gave several formulas to describe the laws in Yin-Yang theory. For example, the changes of Yin and Yang could be represented by following formulas

- $x = X_0 + X_0 \sin(\omega t + \psi)$
- $y = Y_0 - Y_0 \sin(\omega t + \psi)$
- $x + y = 2N$

Similar work was done in five phase and even computers were used to show the stability of the equation group. As the high level of abstractions of Yin and Yang, it is adapted to replace Yin-Yang and five phases by variables. And the relations between Yin and Yang get clearer after represented by mathematic formula. People in the Western world who have basic knowledge of math can easily understand the laws of Yin-Yang in TCM. It somehow improved the TCM. But can we say that the essence of Yin and Yang are just mathematic symbols, they i.e. can be totally replaced by variables. After a detailed discussion with Prof. Wallner in his seminar, I found that this replacement really lost something in Chinese Yin-Yang theory. The lost thing is the nature properties of Yin-Yang. Yin-Yang is the highest abstract property in everything in nature. Everything has two radical aspects which could be distinguished as Yin and Yang. We know what the aspect of Yin is and what the aspect of Yang is according to the TCM theory and Chinese philosophy. But if we replace the Yin and Yang by two mathematic variables, we lose the nature property of Yin and Yang. We could not distinguish a thing by X and Y, namely which aspect of the thing belongs to X and which aspect of the thing belongs to Y. In the couple of heaven and earth, we know heaven belongs to Yang and earth belongs to Yin. But it is difficult to say X is heaven and Y is earth or oppositely.

After strangifying the Yin-Yang by X and Y, we found the limitation of such replacement by Western concept of science and understand Yin and Yang much better than before. The Chinese symbol of Yin and Yang has a specific property which can reflect the nature. With the symbol of Yin-Yang we are closer to nature and more understanding the nature.

The similar process happened in the Eight Diagrams. If we use 0 and 1 to replace the Yin (— —) and the Yang (——), it is easier to operate them on computer but it loses the property of Yin-Yang and the meaning given to the events was lost.

1.8. Conclusions

1. TCM is a science which is different from Western science. TCM constructs the world by imaging which can be called "Constructive Imaging Reality".
2. TCM needs to be understood by Western world and become more efficient. Using Western science in TCM is a way to improve it, but we must be very careful.
3. Strangification in CR is a new methodology which can improve the understanding of TCM. But usually experimental phenomena or literature study should be done firstly while both should be put into the frame of TCM to check the fitness.
4. Putting meridians into Western science, a new unknown knowledge was found in respect to Western medicine and needs to be proved. Using mathematic variables to replace Yin-Yang, the relation between Yin and Yang was clearer but the nature property was lost.
5. After the strangification of Meridian and Yin-Yang, we understood that meridian is a new knowledge in Western science and can hardly be proved only anatomically and Yin-Yang is not just an abstract symbol but has a nature essence inside.

2. LAN FENG-LI: GLOBALIZATION OF TCM: CULTURAL DIFFERENCES BETWEEN TCM AND WESTERN MEDICINE

Lan Feng-Li, Shanghai University of Traditional Chinese Medicine
(Shanghai, P.R. China)

Abstract The thesis discusses cultural differences between traditional Chinese medicine (TCM) and Western medicine from the linguistic and philosophical aspects, the unique values of TCM, and advances some suggestions in the process of globalization of TCM.
Key words Traditional Chinese medicine; Western medicine; cultural differences; globalization

Both transmission of TCM to the West and dissemination of Western medicine in China started in the Ming dynasty (16th-17th centuries). Some missionaries taught and spread religion by practicing Western medicine; meanwhile, they introduced TCM curiously, esp. their own experiences in TCM, to the West. Over 300 years passed by. At present, TCM and Western medicine actually coexist no matter in China or in the West. TCM is not only a special medical system with distinctive national features of China, but is also a medical system for the mankind of the whole world.
Both TCM and Western medicine are "scientific systems of studying life processes of the human being and prevention and treatment of diseases".[1] It is thus clear that they share at least 3 common characters, i.e. the same object: life processes of the human being; the same goal: to prevent and treat diseases; and both are members of "scientific systems". But, TCM bears strong humane characteristics; while Western medicine, esp. modern Western medicine, has typical features of modern Western science. What are the cultural differences between the two medical systems? How do the differences influence the dissemination of TCM in the West, or even globalization of TCM?

2.1. Cultural Differences between TCM and Western Medicine

A leading authority on Chinese herbal medicine, Dr. Yakazu Domei, lists the following differences between TCM and Western Medicine:[2]

---

[1] Xia Zheng-Nong. Sea of Words. Shanghai: Shanghai Dictionary Press, 2002: 2006.
[2] www.tcmhelp.com/Theory/3.htm (9th July 2008).

Chinese Medicine	Western Medicine
Philosophical	Scientific
Synthetic	Analytical
Holistic	Topical
Internal	Surgical
Conformational	Heteropathic
Empirical	Theoretical
Hygienic	Preventive
Individualized	Socialized
Preventive	Bacteriological
Experiential	Experimental
Humoral	Cellular
Subjective	Objective
Natural sources	Synthetic analogy

I will talk about the cultural differences between TCM and Western Medicine from linguistic and philosophical aspects.

2.1.1. Linguistic Differences

"Language is the outcome of culture. Language of a nation is the general reflection of the culture of the nation; but we can also say that language is a part of the culture, and that culture and language have developed together for thousands of years."[3]

2.1.1.1. Ideographic Writing, Phonetic Writing, and Thinking Ways

Ideographic Writing and Thinking Ways of TCM

Chinese characters are the only ideographic writing (as opposed to phonetic writing) which has been preserved for over 3,000 years. As early as in the years of 100-121 A.D., Xu Shen 许慎 of the Eastern Han Dynasty wrote and compiled the first systematic dictionary with complete collection of characters, comprehensive analysis of the shape, pronunciation and meanings as well as scientific arrangement: *The Origin of Chinese Characters* (shuo wen jie zi, "说文解字"). He systematically expounded the theoretical system of the structures of Chinese characters in an all-round way for the first time: the six scripts or the six categories, i.e. *xiangxing* 象形, *zhishi* 指事, *huiyi* 会意, *xingsheng* 形声, *zhuanzhu* 转注 and *jiajie* 假借, and analyzed the structures and meanings of over 9,000 Chinese characters according to the system. Although *The Origin of Chinese*

---

[3] Quoted from A Secondary Source: He Yu-Min. Differences, Perplexity and Selection: A Comparative Study of Chinese Medicine and Western Medicine. Shenyang: Shenyang Press, 1990: 149, 170.

Characters presents and exists in the form of a dictionary, its academic value is far beyond that of the dictionaries in the common sense.

After investigating the authors and their formation times of *The Origin of Chinese Characters* and *Huang Di's Inner Classic,* I have found that it is very possible that the former is influenced by the latter. The following conclusions are reached through comparing and analyzing thinking ways, philosophical conception, and knowledge of human anatomy, disease and treatment in them: (1) The knowledge of TCM contained in *The Origin of Chinese Characters* is in direct line of succession with the *Inner Classic*; (2) The universal and eco-medical thinking ways of "Heaven-Earth-Human being" in them are cut from the same cloth; (3) The theories of qi, yin-yang, and the five phases, the theoretical foundation of the *Inner Classic*, can be traced back to their sources through *The Origin of Chinese Characters* which expounds the original meanings of them by analyzing their structures; (4) *The Origin of Chinese Characters* traces back to characters' origin and original meanings through analyzing their structures, therefore, it is a very helpful and important book to study and read the *Inner Classic*, and to probe into the origin of TCM as well.[4]

Let's take *qi* 气 as an example. *The Origin of Chinese Characters·Qi Section* states that "*Qi* refers to thin, floating clouds. The character 气 is a pictographic character."[5] The character 气 in *Jia Gu Wen* 甲骨文, the inscriptions on bones or tortoise shells of the Shang Dynasty (c. 16th-11th century B.C.), was written as "川", which resembles air current, evaporating and rising, whose image is just like cloud, will disappear very soon and become invisible. Therefore, *qi* is invisible and formless, exists everywhere, can be gathered into a form, for instance, *qi* can be condensed into water. *Qi* at this moment referred to air or vapor.

Soon afterwards, the *qi* which surrounds and congests the space of the human being was abstracted into the *qi* which bears a material meaning in philosophical sense. Philosophers of materialism of the Spring Autumn and Warring States Period (770-221B.C.) believed that *qi* is the basic material constituting the world, and that everything in the universe comes into being by the movement and mutation of *qi*. For example, *Book of Changes • Section Xi Ci,* (Zhou Yi • Xi Ci, "周易•系辞") states that "everything is transformed and generated by the enshrouding [qi] of the heaven and earth".

Later on, ancient Chinese medical experts introduced "*qi*" into the medical field at the right moment. And then, "*qi*" became a medium or bridge between the natural philosophy of the pre-Qin days (i.e. before 221 B.C. when the First Emperor of Qin united China) and Chinese medicine. The concept of "*qi*" gradually formed in TCM.

---

[4] Lan Feng-Li. *Influence of Huang Di's Inner Classic on the Origin of Chinese Character.* Chinese Journal of Medical History, 2006 (2).
[5] Written by Xu Shen [Han], Annotated by Duan Yu-Cai [Qing]. The Origin of Chinese Characters with Annotations. Shanghai: Shnaghai Ancient Books Press, 1988: 20.

In the time of *Huangdi's Inner Classic*, "*qi*" is regarded not only as the basic material constituting the world, but also as the basic material constituting the human being which can be transformed into blood, essence, and body fluid, etc., and the normal functional activities of the life which is governed by "qi" is known as *Shen* or spirit.[6]

It is thus evident that *the shape of a Chinese character is directly related to its meaning, and both integrate into a unity. The formation of a Chinese character, an organic whole of the shape and the meaning, is one-step made following the rule of nature, reflecting the direct communication between and integration of the subject and the object.* The formation also implies an important thinking way, i.e. *thinking in terms of images*. Integration of the subject and the object is a thread running through the Chinese traditional culture and science, on the basis of which the unification of the Heaven and Human being (tian ren he yi, 天人合一) constitutes the foundation of the Chinese traditional culture and sciences. Thinking in terms of images is a traditional thinking way of the Chinese nation, and whose process, methods, and rules make up *the thinking in terms of images and reasoning from analogy (qu xiang bi lei,* 取象比类*)*, the framework of the Chinese traditional culture and sciences.

Developed on the basis of the ideographic writing, Chinese characters and their meanings are quite stable and conservative, which greatly promotes the development of the thinking in terms of images and reasoning from analogy of ancient TCM experts. Then such a thinking way was set up in the *Huang Di's Inner Classic* and has greatly influenced TCM experts of the later generations.

The ideographic writings of yin-yang 阴阳, *wu xing, or five phases* 五行, *jing or essence* 精, and *qi*, the extensive analogical and abundant imagery thinking examples in the *Huang Di's Inner Classic*, and criticism, proofreading, annotations for characters from the aspects of the "shape", "pronunciation", and "meaning" in the ancient medical classics made in the Ming (1368-1644 A.D.) and Qing Dynasties (1644-1911 A.D.), all demonstrate the far-reaching influences of the ideographic thinking way on the development of TCM.

Phonetic Writing, and Thinking Ways of Western Medicine

Phonetic writing (as opposed to ideographic writing) is the most common writing in the world. English, German, French, Spanish, Portuguese, etc. are all phonetic writing, but are different languages composed by the same Latin alphabet. Let's take English as a case in point.

The shapes of the English words are directly related to the pronunciations, but have nothing to do with the meanings or the external images of concrete things. That is to say, in phonetic writing, the shape is separate and independent from

---

[6] Lan Feng-li. The Origin of *Qi*, *Yin-Yang* and *Wu Xing* as Chinese Medical Concepts and Their Translation. Forthcoming, 2008.

the meaning, and the meaning comes from man-made prescript outside the shape, which indicates that the formation of a word of the phonetic writing is composed of two steps: first, building its shape (spelling of alphabets); second, defining its meaning (linguistic rules or grammar). The understanding of the meanings of words is based on the sense of hearing, thus jumping out the thinking frame of the visual sense of the concrete images of things, then providing a bigger possibility for logic thinking based on the abstraction, finally forming thinking traditions of abstract inference, conceptual thinking, categorization, and trying to make an objective judgment to the world.

This is really indeed the case. *The formation of phonetic writing reflects its two important characteristics: tool (alphabet) and abstraction (linguistic rules).* Every tool is made to have a certain function according to human beings' specific aim or intention, thus becoming a medium of connection between human beings and the nature, and so interrupting the natural direct communication between them. Tool plays a vital role in the Western culture, esp. in the natural sciences, where it is standardized and systematized, and the experimental research approach characterized by the use of various tools is set up. *Actually, the alphabet is the mother of various tools.* The thinking way corresponding to the experimental research approach is abstraction. *The rule of abstraction is logic, while linguistic rules or grammar is an embryonic form of logic.*[7]

The emergence of tool reflects the relationship between the subject and the object, i.e., the separation and opposition of them (man remakes the nature). The abstraction pays more attention to being analytical, logical, and restricts imagination. The tool and abstraction become the foundation of the Western culture and sciences and of the natural sciences (including the Western medicine) in particular. The Western natural sciences manifest in two opposite ways or two edges, which have been realized by more and more people as time goes by. The two edges lie in that environmental pollution and ecological imbalance, the repay of the nature to the human beings, always accompany the process of human conquering and remaking nature. As regards to the Western medicine, the two edges lie in that severe side effects, drug resistance, and effect being temporary always accompany the notable therapeutic effects.

2.1.1.2. Chinese Medical Terminology and Western Medical Terminology

Undoubtedly, no matter the language of TCM or the language of Western medicine is a kind of technical language. Modern terminologists define a "technical language" as a form of any given language that is used by people involved in a special field and that has a "terminology", i.e., a set of expressions not used in

---

[7] Wang Zhen-Hua. Theoretical Difference between TCM and Western Medicine on the Basis of Linguistics: Modernization of TCM. China Journal of Traditional Chinese Medicine. 2001: 16 (6): 5.

the common language or, as is often the case, expressions that are used in a different or more specific way than in the common language.

A popular misconception about technical terms is that they are words used *exclusively* by specialists. *In actual fact, technical terms in most disciplines largely, if not mostly, come from the common language.* Any language only has a certain number of words, and new terms are usually combinations of existing lexical items. Many terms are completely indistinguishable in form from expressions in the common language although they are more specific in meaning. The process whereby common language expressions are given more specific or metaphorical meanings in the technical contexts is called "terminologization". *The modern terminological observation that technical terms are largely derived from the common language is reflected clearly both in TCM and Western medicine.* Those acquainted with the language of TCM are aware that most of the characters they come across in Chinese medical texts are used in the common language. And most of the Western medical terms are combinations of morphemes of Latin or Greek. Actually, about 10,000 Latin or Greek words came into English during the Renaissance Period and finally became a part of English vocabulary.

Actually, both TCM terminology and Western medical terminology can be classified into three levels: (1) words and expressions for everyday use; (2) specialized terms of their own; and (3) original terms of their own.

Three Levels of Chinese Medical Terminology

Both Dr. Wiseman and Prof. Unschuld advocated classifying the basic Chinese medical terminology into two categories: one comprises of words and expressions for everyday use, e.g., 头 head, 脚 foot, 胸 chest, 腹 abdomen, 心 heart, 肝 liver, 血 blood; the other is composed of specialized TCM terms extended from the common language and formed through metaphor or analogy, e.g., 窍 orifice, 穴 point or hole, 正 upright, 邪 evil, 营 nutrient, 卫 defense, 命门 life gate, 督脉 the governing vessel, 三焦 triple passage or triple burner or triple energizer.[8] [Note: The character 焦, as a common character, does mean "burnt" or "charred", but as a medical term, it means "passage or space within the body" that is well explained in some specialized Chinese dictionaries.]

According to my understanding of Chinese medical terminology, esp. of *the Origin of Chinese Characters*, I think that Chinese medical terminology can be classified into 3 levels. The first level is made up of *words and expressions from the common language*, e.g., some body parts like 心 heart, 肝 liver, 脾 spleen, 肺 lungs, 肾 kidneys, 鼻 nose, 目 eyes, 耳 ears, 头 head, 脚 foot, 胸 chest, 腹 abdomen, 血 blood; some disease names like 霍乱 cholera, 麻疹 measles, 麻风 leprosy, 疟疾 malaria, 癫痫 epilepsy; some climatic pathogenic factors like 风

---

[8] Wiseman, Nigel. Translation and Transmission of Chinese Medicine in the West. Medicine and Philosophy. 2001, 22 (7): 51-54.

wind, 寒 cold, 湿 dampness, 燥 dryness, 火 fire; some symptoms like 发热 fever, 头痛 headache, 痛 pain, 咳嗽 cough, 心悸 palpitation, 健忘 forgetfulness, 头晕目眩 dizziness, 呕吐 vomiting, 恶心 nausea, 泄泻 diarrhea, 便秘 (不更衣) constipation. The second level constitutes *specialized Chinese medical terms from daily words and expressions formed through metaphor or analogy*, e.g., 藏 depots or viscera, 府 palaces or bowels, 经 meridian or channel, 络 collateral or network vessel, 窍 orifice, 穴 point or hole, 正 upright, 邪 evil, 营 nutrient, 卫 defense, 督脉 the governing vessel, 任脉 the controlling vessel, 三焦 the triple energizer or *san jiao*, 命门 life gate, etc. *which usually bear historical, cultural, and medical values at the same time.* The third level comprises of *original Chinese medical terms*, e.g., *some pictophonetic characters* such as 疝, 疽, 痈, 疡, 痔, 瘘, 痹, etc. in *The Origin of Chinese Characters • Disease Section*.

Three Levels of Western Medical Terminology

Dr. Wiseman roughly classified the Western medical terminology into 3 levels and distinguished them as well. The first level constitutes *borrowings from the common language*, e.g., fever, chill, cough, cold, hiccough, headache, pain, tenderness, soreness, palpitations, bleeding, hot flushes, forgetfulness, dizziness, vomiting, blindness, jaundice, deafness, nausea, emaciation, diarrhea, constipation, goiter, sores, corn, sty, boil, measles, mumps, and fracture. These words, commonly used by doctors, are known to all speakers and denote conditions that can be identified by most normal adults. The second level comprises *terms devised by modern medicine to describe certain technical concepts*: conjunctivitis, anemia, hypertension, paranasal sinusitis, trichomoniasis, arteriosclerosis, optic atrophy, hyperchlorhydria, coronary thrombosis, glomerulonephritis hematoma, cerebrovascular ischemia. Although some of these words (such as anemia, hypertension and conjunctivitis) may be familiar to and even used by non-experts, the conditions they denote cannot be diagnosed by the non-experts with the medical precision. These terms *reflect knowledge that lies at a long distance from lay understanding.* Between these two levels is *a third comprising term of medical origin* that do not require any specialist knowledge or instrumentation to understand or identify, e.g., enuresis, lochia, pharynx, larynx, dysphagia, strangury, scrofula, tumor, fistula, miliaria, macule, papule, and diphtheria.[9]

I think that the terms of the first level are actually from *words and expressions for everyday use*, that of the second level are *specialized terms of Western medicine*, and that of the third level are *original terms of Western medicine*.

---

[9] Wiseman, Nigel. The Translation of Chinese Medical Terminology. English-Chinese & Chinese-English Dictionary of Chinese Medicine, Changsha: Hunan Science and Technology Press, 1996: 67.

Remarks

In the course of transmission and exchange of medical cultures, linguistic contact is a forerunner of the contact of different medical cultures. Language, an essential medium, is the carrier of the medical knowledge. The transmission and exchange between different medical cultures will first manifest in the terminology. The foreign terminology comes to be the "envoy" of the different medical cultures. Generally speaking, a foreign medical culture is introduced and disseminated by translating the foreign medical terminology. The translated terminology gradually integrates into the native language, finally becomes an organic part of the mainstream medical culture of the nation proper.

The history of translation and dissemination of Western medicine in China shows that the Western medical terminology and culture are very closely associated with each other, just like the shadow following the person. It also took a very long time for the formation of standard Chinese translation of Western medical terminology in China. In the early stage of translation and dissemination of Western medicine in China, for example, translation of the term "scarlet fever" had been very confusing, which had many different translations such as 红热症, 红疹, 疹子热病, 痧病, 花红热症, 猩红热, etc.

It can be seen from the history and reality of translating Western medicine into Chinese that the first and third levels of the Chinese medical terms have been successfully used to express Western medical knowledge, and that using the second level of Chinese medical terms, which carry the most distinctive TCM knowledge, to translate specialized terms of Western medicine, has produced serious confusions or even mistakes. Here are two examples:

(1) Translating "typhoid" into 伤寒 Typhoid refers to "infection of the intestine caused by Salmonella typhi in food and water"[10], manifesting in fever, diarrhea, even bloody stool; while 伤寒 is a specialized Chinese medical term, bears two meanings in TCM: in a broad sense, 伤寒, cold-induced disease, is a general term for various externally contracted febrile diseases, as stated in the Plain Questions·Discourse on Febrile Diseases (su wen·re lun, "素问•热论") "今夫热病者, 皆伤寒之类也"; in a narrow sense, 伤寒, cold affection, refers to a condition caused by cold, manifesting in chills and fevers, absence of sweating, headache, floating and tense pulse, as stated in the Classic of Difficult Issues (nan jing, "难经·五十八难" "伤寒有五 : 有中风, 有伤寒, 有湿温, 有热病, 有温病, 其所苦各不同". Later on, some translators rendered 伤寒 in Chinese medicine back into "typhoid". Such a translation has confused the differences between "typhoid" in Western medicine and 伤寒 in Chinese medicine, thus causing misunderstanding or even misleading the readers.

---

[10] Collin, P.H. Dictionary of Medicine. Beijing: Foreign Language Teaching and Research Press, 2001: 613, 571.

(2) Translating "surgery" into 外科学 Surgery refers to "treatment of a disease or disorder which requires an operation to cut into or to remove or to manipulate tissue or organs or parts"[11]; while 外科学 in TCM refers to a specialty which studies the causes, pathogenesis, and treatments of the diseases on the body surface.[12] Many TCM undergraduates or even doctorate candidates, and some translators translate 外科学 in TCM into "Surgery". Actually, 外科学 in TCM should be translated into "external medicine" for the real "surgery" in TCM declined long ago since Hua Tuo died in 208 A.D.

We should draw some lessons from the above mentioned translation examples that the second level of Western medical terms should not be used to translate and express the specialized Chinese medical terms. For example, although 风火眼 in TCM and "acute conjunctivitis" in Western medicine actually refer to the same disease, it is ill-advised to translate 风火眼 into "acute conjunctivitis" for such a translation must confuse cultural differences between the two medical systems, and fail to produce such association of the cause (pathogenic wind-fire) and therapeutic method (coursing wind and clearing fire) with the translation "acute conjunctivitis", thus destroying the independency, wholeness and systematicness of the theoretical system of TCM.

An interesting issue to be addressed is that some disease names in the *Plain Questions (su wen)* may be of foreign origin. Here are some examples: *li lai* 疠癞: 疠, whose ancient pronunciation is *ljadh* or *rjats*, and 癞, whose ancient pronunciation is *ladh* or *rats*, the initial consonants come closer to those of the three most popular ancient European terms for *leprosy*, one might speculate about an association of *li* and *lai* with *leuke, lepra, and e-lephantiasis*; *huo luan* 霍乱, the compound *huo luan* does not correspond to the graphic structure of the vast majority of ancient Chinese disease terms, while its ancient pronunciation **hwak* luan* was formed to reflect in ancient Chinese the sound of the term *cholera* used along the travel routes from regions where the Greek term was in use to the Far East to designate a particularly violent type of diarrhea; *fei xiao* 肺消, whose ancient pronunciation is **phjats*sjaw,* literally "lung wasting", could be a rendering into Chinese of the ancient Greek term *phtisis* or lung *phtisis*, which has exactly the same meaning; xiao ke 消渴, wasting/melting and thirst, a label used to this day for diabetes, is a compound ideally suited to signify two obvious symptoms of the disease. An identical meaning was expressed in European antiquity by Aretaios of Cappadochia.[13] Is it purely coincidental? Or there existed medical cultural exchange between the East and the West around the Zhou Dy-

---

[11] Collin, P.H. Dictionary of Medicine. Beijing: Foreign Language Teaching and Research Press, 2001: 613, 571.
[12] Li Jing-Wei, et al. A Concise Dictionary of Chinese Medicine. Beijing: China Press of Traditional Chinese Medicine: 301.
[13] Unschuld, Paul U. Huang Di Nei Jing Su Wen: Nature, Knowledge, Imagery in An Ancient Chinese Medical Text. Berkeley: University of California Press, 2003: 203-204.

nasty (C.1100-256B.C.)? Anyway, these terms all came out far before the modern Western medicine and should be regarded as the terms of the first level. The above understanding further provides etymological evidence when translating 疠癞, 霍乱, 肺消, 消渴 into leprosy, cholera, lung wasting, wasting and thirst respectively.

2.1.1.3. Medical Classical Chinese and Medical English

First of all, let's look at the two paragraphs about the origin of human life both from the angle of genetics in TCM and Western medicine respectively:
(1) "人生于地, 悬命于天, 天地合气, 命之曰人. 人能应四时者,
天地为之父母" („素问•宝命全形论").
Translation: Man is born on the earth, hanging his life to the heaven. The union of celestial qi and terrestrial qi make up a man. Man can adapt himself to the seasons for the Heaven and Earth are his parents. (Plain Questions·Discourse on Protecting Life and Preserving Physical Appearance)
(2) "Man is metazoon, triploblastic, chordale, vertebrate, pentadactyle, mammalian, eutherian, primate… The outlines of each of his principal system of organs may be traced back, like those of other mammals, to the fishes." (L.A.B.-orradaile)
(译文：人属于后生动物, 系五趾, 三胚层高级动物, 属脊索动物门,
脊椎动物亚门, 哺乳纲, 灵长目…象其它哺乳动物一样,
他的每一个器官系统的轮廓可以追溯到鱼类。)[14]

It is thus clear that the Chinese language of the first paragraph is very elegant and beautiful, is composed of four-character or six-character sentences like a poem or a prose, thus pertaining to classical style and bearing some characteristics of humane studies; while the English language of the second paragraph is very rigorous and precise, comprises of technical terms, thus pertaining to technical style and bearing typical features of Western science.

It is well known that the core knowledge of TCM comes from the ancient medical texts in classical style of writing. In fact, the TCM language has been set to "classical style of writing" since the era of *Huang Di's Inner Classic*. Medical classical Chinese is one of "classical styles of writing", a literary style of writing. TCM terminology is polysemous and ambiguous, and medical classical Chinese is very succinct in style and rich in figures of speech, so the meanings of TCM language tend to be ambiguous and initiate contentions among different schools. The theoretical framework of TCM is extraordinary stable and has almost no breakthrough since *Huang Di's Inner Classic, Classic of Difficult Issues, Shen Nong's Classic of Materia Medica*, and *Treatise on Cold-Induced and Miscellaneous Diseases* came out several thousands of years ago. TCM has been

---

[14] Hou Wei-Rui. English Styles of Writing. Shanghai: Shanghai Foreign Language Education Press, 1988: 278.

paying excessive attention to wording since the era of the *Inner Classic*, and textual criticism, exegetical studies and annotations of ancient medical classics has been an important academic field of study in TCM up till now, thus reflecting its characteristics of humane and social studies.

As regards to Western medicine, esp. modern Western medicine, it is no doubt that it has been developing with amazing speed and has made many breakthroughs and astonishing achievements in the 19th-21st centuries. "The main reason that the natural sciences have developed more mature than the social sciences is that most of the natural sciences have liberated themselves from the wording disputations and that paying excessive attention to wording has been still spreading unchecked in various ways in the social sciences no matter in the past or nowadays".[15]

2.1.2. Philosophical Differences

Philosophy, the core of culture and the theoretical thinking of the top level, has been guiding the development of medicine and other sciences. Traditional Western thinking mode is known as analytical thinking, causal thinking, or conceptual thinking[16], on the basis of which the mechanism, reductionism, dichotomy formed and greatly promoted the development of Western medicine. Surgery and organ transplantation medicine have developed on the basis of the mechanism which views the human body as a "machine". On the basis of reductionist ideology or reductionism that is, it seeks to understand a system by breaking it down into its constituent parts, experimental physiology and cellular biology were founded in the 19th century and molecular biology was founded in the 20th century; influenced by such a thinking, the Western medicine has studied various systems and organs of the body down to cell, to molecule, and to gene in the recent 2 centuries, and constructed a series branches of learning of basic medicine, thus forming the so-called "scientific" Western medicine. Dichotomy, philosophy of a division into two opposite parts: A and Non-A , indicates the separation of the subject and object, of the nature and human being, of the time and space, of the body and mind, of the ontology and epistemology, and so and so forth, guides the treating principle of Western medicine as well which treats a condition using drugs which produce opposite symptoms to those of the condition.

---

[15] Quoted from A Secondary Source: He Yu-Min. Differences, Perplexity and Selection: A Comparative Study of Chinese Medicine and Western Medicine. Shenyang: Shenyang Press, 1990: 149, 170.

[16] Fang Ke-Li. A Fusion of Chinese and Western Cultures and Modern Transformation of Chinese Philosophy. Beijing: Commercial Press, 2003: 140-143.

Traditional Chinese thinking mode is known as correlative thinking[17], which originated in the *Book of Changes* and is mainly characterized by explaining dynamic life processes by opposing and complementing as the Yin-Yang Diaphragm suggests. The correlative thinking sees everything in the universe as interdependent and interactive. In TCM, the correlative thinking manifests itself concretely in the yin-yang theory, the five-phase theory, and the visceral image theory, the vessel theory, etc., which evolved in the way of following the features of the heaven and earth (nature) to the human being from concrete to abstract, from structure to function. In TCM, disease is regarded as the result of imbalance or disharmony of yin and yang, and the goal of TCM treatment is to restore the balance for each individual under his or her own unique environment.

Actually, correlative thinking mode of Eastern tradition and causal thinking mode of Western tradition depend on each other and complement to each other, to some extent oppose to each other. More and more scholars in the West have recognized this point.

Compared to the Western philosophical thinking mode, traditional Chinese philosophical thinking mode is not inferior at all, but can be a perfect complement to the Western philosophical thinking. The two traditions should understand each other, respect each other. Only in this way, each tradition can understand its own culture more thoroughly; the two traditions can promote each other and develop together.

2.2. Unique Values of TCM

2.2.1. Unique Value of TCM Theories

Most of traditional medical systems declined long ago. But TCM has aroused attention and studies of the world medical circle. What is the reason? Is it due to Chinese medicinals or acupuncture or thousands of years of clinical experiences? No, it is not really the case. The key lies in that TCM has a set of systematic, macrocosmic theory which can effectively guide clinical practice, challenge or even overcome baffling problems of the world medical circle. For example, SARS (Severe Acute Respiratory Syndrome) was so successfully treated in China according to the Warm Disease Theory during its attack in 2003 that experts of World Health Organization (WHO) highly appraised the effects and suggested to improve such clinical experiences to a level of routine treatment; Prof. Deng Tie-Tao (邓铁涛) successfully treated many stubborn diseases such as gravis myoasthenia, atrophic gastritis, hepatitis, cirrhosis, aplastic anemia, lupus erythematosus, etc. according to the Spleen-Stomach Theory; many cases with high fever who failed to respond to antibiotics or antipyretics were successfully

---

[17] Fang Ke-Li. A Fusion of Chinese and Western Cultures and Modern Transformation of Chinese Philosophy. Beijing: Commercial Press, 2003: 140-143.

cured according to the Theory of Sweet and Warm Medicinals Being Capable of Relieving High Fever.

TCM theories are unique in Chinese sciences and culture and are based on the correlative thinking and holism, therefore, reductionist methodology of the Western scientific approach is not applicable for the study of TCM. For example, White Tiger Decoction is a famous formula for relieving high fever. But Western pharmacological studies found that each ingredient of the formula did not show any effect in relieving fever in experimental animals, which indicates that the reductionist methodology does not work in traditional Chinese pharmacological studies and that traditional Chinese pharmacological studies can not break away from the systematic theory and clinical practice of TCM.

Deng Tie-Tao said, "Microcosmic is a scientific approach, macrocosmic is also a scientific approach. Scientific studies can be done not only based on microcosmic approach, but also can be done on the basis of macrocosmic approach of TCM".[18] "TCM and Western medicine should not repel each other but should complement each other. Integration of microcosmic and macrocosmic approaches will produce a more profound theory, and achieve a better therapeutic effect. This is the developmental orientation of post-modern sciences".[19]

2.2.2. Distinctive Glamour of TCM Therapeutics

TCM has survived the challenge of Western medicine and even advanced to some extent in the 20th-21st centuries mainly for it can effectively treat many diseases.

It is well known that most of gynecological disorders such as menstrual disorders, infertility, climacteric syndrome, etc. can be successfully treated by TCM while Western medicine can only provide hormone and surgical operation.

As regards to emergency treatments, *Da Chai Hu* Decoction recorded in *Treatise on Cold-Induced Diseases* (*Shang han lun*, "伤寒论") is remarkably effective in treating acute pancreasitis, *Da Jian Zhong* Decoction recorded in *Synopsis of the Golden Chamber* (*Jin Kui Yao Lue*, "金匮要略") remarkably effective in treating paralytic intestinal obstruction, puncturing the *Si Feng* points (EX-UE10) remarkably effective in treating intestinal obstruction due to round worms, and so and so forth.

Both history and reality have proved that lemology of TCM also has its own distinctive glamour. TCM has successfully resolved prevention and treatment of various infectious diseases, esp. infectious diseases caused by various viruses, such as encephalitis B, measles complicated with pneumonia, SARS, etc.

---

[18] Bian Shi Ji (A Collection of Distinguished TCM Experts' Papers). Beijing: China Press of Traditional Chinese Medicine, 2001: 4.
[19] Deng Tie-Tao. Correctly Understanding Chinese Medicine. China Newspaper of Chinese Medicine. 2003 (2): 17.

Besides, TCM can also successfully deal with functional disorders of the nervous, endocrine, and immune systems, diseases of undetermined causes, diseases of complicated causes and pathomechanism, diseases in chronic or recovery stage, and disease prevention and health preservation based on pattern identification and treatment.

2.2.3. Doctor's Cardinal Humane Care to Patient (medical morality): Different Relationship between Doctor and Patient

In TCM culture, medicine is a kind of benevolent skill, a doctor should be benevolent to the patients, cultivate his morality, love his career, study diligently, train hard, be conscientious, responsible, modest and prudent, respect his colleagues, which fully reflect in Sun Simiao's *Medical Morality* (or A great doctor should be expert in medical skills and sincere to the patients, da yi jing cheng, "大医精诚", the preface of the *Invaluable Prescriptions for Emergencies*, bei ji qian jin yao fang, "备急千金要方"; Sun Si-Miao, 541 or 581~682, a great doctor of the Tang Dynasty).

Sun Si-Miao said, "When the well-qualified doctors treat patients, they should be calm and concentrated without any desire or avarice. First of all, they should have great sympathy for the patients and then be determined to save people from the suffering. When patients come to ask for help, they should not treat them differently by seeing whether they are rich or poor, old or young, beautiful or ugly, enemy or friend, Chinese or foreigner, foolish or wise. They should treat all the patients like their close relatives. When treating patients, they should not think over and over for themselves and pay too much attention to the protection of their own lives. Being qualified doctors, they should regard the patients' suffering as their own and have deep sympathy for them. They should not try to avoid danger if being confronted with it. No matter in daytime or night, winter or summer, no matter they are hungry or thirsty, tired or exhausted, they should treat or save patients heart and soul without any delay or worrying about personal gains or losses. Only by so doing can they become great doctors for people".

2.3. Globalization of TCM: Opportunity and Challenge

We have to face such a stern reality: Information in English accounted for over 80% of the total information stored in the computers of the world; databases owned by U.S.A. made up over 70% of the globe;[20] the statistics of the United Nations showed that of all the original documents 80% were in English and less than 1% in Chinese; there existed great deficit in the cultural exchange: the

---

[20] Yu Ke-Ping. Globalization: Westernization or Chinesization. Beijing: Social Sciences Academic Press, 2002: 4-256.

works translated from Western languages into Chinese were about 50 to 100 times of the works translated from Chinese into Western languages.[21]

Does globalization mean Westernization, Easternization or similarization or even uniformation? No, globalization should be pluralization. Almost everybody has traveling experience. As a traveler, everyone would like to see something, some place, and some people with distinctive, specialized, and local features. If everywhere is the same someday in the future, the world will be very boring. This is the same as the culture. Standing on the international academic platform, reviewing the history of human beings fighting against diseases, preserving health and prolonging life, we have to realize that TCM is a real gem worth to cherish and to carry on in the unending quest for human health and a long life.

2.3.1. Standardize Academic Language of TCM

We have to establish the coordinate rules of TCM before opening a dialogue for the cultural exchange of TCM with outside world. First of all, we should strengthen the studies on the standardization of academic language of TCM in the process of translating and introducing TCM works to the West. As Shigeru Omi said, *"Science and civilization have developed because of language. Likewise, traditional medicine has been developing for thousands of years with its own set of terms. [...] Although traditional medicine can be defined with indigenous characters, its terminology should be standardized for modern usage. International standard terminology will greatly expedite scientific communications in traditional societies. It is the very first step towards the globalization of traditional medicine."*[22]

We should systematize the basic theories, fundamental propositions, core concepts, essential terminology and key words of TCM, make them conformable to each other, then expound and make a comment on them in a rationale way for the purpose of avoiding misunderstanding or misleading the readers in the process of outputting TCM.

We should interpret Chinese medical classics thoroughly with plentiful clinical experiences and modern research results, not just explain the classics word for word.

It is very important to study the differences between TCM in China (original TCM) and the TCM transmitted in the West in order to learn from each other, bridge the gap and make TCM better known, studied, and appreciated for many years to come no matter in China or in the West.

---

[21] Wang Yue-Chuan. Discovering the East. Beijing: Beijing Library Press, 2003: 29.
[22] WHO Western Pacific Region. WHO International Standard Terminologies on Traditional Medicine in the Western Pacific Region. Forward. 2007.

2.3.2. Popularize TCM Knowledge Worldwide

It is very important to popularize medical knowledge to the common people, esp. the knowledge of TCM to the young people, in order to let them know the advantages and disadvantages of TCM and Western medicine. Encourage them to see more TCM. According to Wu Yi's (吴仪, Vice Primer of the Government of China) talk on the development of TCM, TCM knowledge in popular language will be written into textbooks of primary and middle schools in China in the near future. The role and position of TCM in the health care system of China is vital in the process of spreading it worldwide.

A cooperation group, which is composed of Chinese and Western scholars of the related fields, should be organized in order to translate and introduce real TCM in a more attractive, readable and "digestive" way in different levels to the corresponding intended readers. For example, the books should be translated or written in a popular style and good language for the common people; for practitioners of TCM, TCM academic language, which preserves the systematicness, independency, and wholeness of the theoretical system of TCM, should be strictly applied; for experts of medical history, the translation should preserve the cultural, historical, and medical values of the original texts; for doctors or researchers of Western medicine, the text should contain more modern research results, or more "evidence-based"; etc.

2.3.3. Keep Characteristics of TCM and Bring Them into Full Play

As we all know, individualized treatment based on pattern identification is one of the basic characteristics and great vitality of TCM. Therefore, we should study the essence and connotations of pattern identification and treatment; try to discover the relationship among patterns in TCM and physio-chemical indexes, diseases in modern Western medicine; apply modern technology to check the therapeutic effects of TCM, or even invent some new apparatus in the light of TCM theory to check the effects; set up or found a system in the light of TCM theory to assess, approve, and verify research projects or modern studies of TCM.

In the context of globalization, the differences of TCM from Western medicine should be highlighted in almost all aspects. For example, the appearance and inner design of the TCM clinics or hospitals should reflect TCM cultural features such as by using yin-yang diaphragm, popularizing the knowledge of the prevention and treatment of common diseases, of health preservation in the different seasons, and caring more patients' needs, etc. The theory related to health preservation should be studied and TCM hospitals or clinics should provide consultant service for healthy or sub-healthy people on disease prevention and health preservation

2.3.4. Train More Elites of TCM in the Traditional Way

Many modern distinguished practitioners of TCM like Shi Jinmo 施今墨, Jiang Chunhua 姜春华, Pu Fuzhou 蒲辅周, Yue Meizhong 岳美中, Zhu Weiju 祝味菊, Deng Tietao 邓铁涛, Ren Jixue 任继学, and so and so forth, had a solid foundation of TCM, and were very creative no matter in theory or practice. Their medical attainments and skills in diagnosing and treating diseases are a wonderful integration of personal disposition, cultural accomplishments, clinical experiences, and expression of personal academic ideas. We should attach great importance to the study of these distinguished TCM experts in order to discover the way of their innovation and success both in the theoretical and clinical explorations.

More practitioners or elites of TCM should be trained in the traditional way. For example, Shandong University of TCM painstakingly chooses about 20 students every year to be trained in a more traditional way for successive 7 years: less hours in Western medicine and more hours in TCM; no hours in English and more hours in TCM classics; learn to recognize, collect, prepare, and process Chinese medicinals; learn to make different preparation forms of Chinese medicine like pill, powder, extract; learn almost all available therapies of TCM including tuina, acupuncture, moxibustion, herbal remedies; follow certain doctors or teachers to learn skills; etc.

TCM is a great treasure house of Chinese culture, and an important component part of the world civilization. Eastern culture and Western culture should be set to equal status, and both are the common spiritual wealth of the human being. As Confucius said, "Men of noble character can be harmonious but different". I do hope TCM and Western medicine can harmoniously coexist worldwide to contribute together to the human health and well-being.

3. GÜNTER GUNIA: DEVELOPMENT AND POSSIBILITIES OF TCM

Günter Gunia
University of Potsdam

My interest in acupuncture began in 1990. I could never have imagined breaking with my medical technique at this time. Nevertheless, it was already part of my holistic medical vision through which I was constantly obliged to feel personally responsible for understanding and for the well-being of my patients. So, my fascination by a report from a colleague who had visited a lecture on acupuncture at the medical faculty of the University of Hanover was hardly a coincidence: People who had spent many years going from doctor to doctor and out-patients' ward to clinic experienced understanding for the first time and relief if not healing and the solution to their problems through acupuncture. Back then I was invited to weekend courses in acupuncture regularly. However, the subject matter, and the fact that the courses were fragmented on the weekends, failed to awaken my interest. A pharmaceuticals representative once gave me a present picture book on ear acupuncture but despite intensive engagement with this book, I found no access to the theme. My colleague's experience with the acupuncture lecture at the university clinic reminded me how many chronically ill patients I had treated who had received similar specialist doctors' and special clinic diagnoses as described in the acupuncture lecture. I now saw the chance to satisfy these patients through acupuncture. Nothing could have been worse than to live with complaints and pain and to repeatedly hear from doctors how healthy one was or that nothing more could be done for them. Based on the results of the TCM lecture, the problem did not lie with the patients but with us doctors who believe that there is only one medicine. If we have to tell our patients that no form of treatment is effective for them or that no therapy is possible, we are often only demonstrating our own limitations. The fewest among us admit this to themselves or their patients. Economic arguments have come into play today. Only those treatments which one administers oneself can insure one's existence. Furthermore, it is economically more attractive to offer chronically ill patients western-oriented treatments than to cure them with far-eastern methods. The danger in Chinese medicine is that it helps. Chronically ill patients ensure the health industry's income. The healthy rheumatic, asthmatic or neurodermetic no longer visits a doctor as often and doesn't take medication or use ointments. It can not be ruled out that medication even supports chronic illness. They certainly also help but are possibly addictive and bind us to our illnesses. Chinese medicine and other complimentary medicines do not encumber the organism with chemicals or toxins. It focuses on the basic perturbance of the organs and utilises the body's own resources without restriction to somatic aspects. Body, soul, and mind are brought into balance. We know today through psychoneuroimmunology how important socio-psychological considerations are, without respecting the fact that TCM was already incorporating such aspects many thousands of years ago. It is interesting to see that TCM is not only made use of by alternatively-oriented people, but increasingly by critical, health-oriented people from leading positions or due to their academic studies. Interest in alternative healing methods is not only driven by the strain of suffering or disappointing experiences with western medicine but above all by a new health awareness with interest in prevention and Salutogenesis. It is less and less about satisfying basic needs and increasingly about feeling good and quality of life. The future of ageing also brings duties to provide quality to the later years of life. This involves not only movement, nutrition and the avoidance of toxins but also constant examination of the energy balance (resources). The older person can compensate for failings in performance and physical or emotional perturbances with TCM in the same way in which an executive or other person under high psycho-intellectual strain can reconstitute or improve performance through energy balance with Chinese medicine. Ageing is not inevitably connected with restrictions on quality of life or health. The Employers Federation recognised many years ago how important active health maintenance will be in the work phase and in the following retirement phase. A clear reduction in health costs is a positive effect of maintaining health in old age. My experience has shown that organic and functional perturbances can be controlled by acupuncture well after the 90th year of life and so, joy in life can be maintained in the sunset years. As well as life's later years, the beginning of life also finds its correlation to TCM. Fertility issues in women and men are often a great problem for young couples who wish to fulfil their family planning. TCM can also remove organic, functional, hormonal obstacles to help establish the happy family. Should problems occur during pregnancy, such as nausea omitting in early pregnancy, badly positioned foetus, or ante-natal gestosis or many other health problems such as colds and rheumatic illness these can of course be treated without chemicals or burden through Chinese medicine without harming mother or child. Of course the birth can be steered and induced by acupuncture. And the new life can also benefit from acupuncture as soon as it has arrived: Feeding, digestive and sleep problems can be treated in infants by sticking seed plasters in the ear as all children's' illnesses can be healed thereafter. Acupuncture can influence all organs and bodily functions via the vegetative nervous system without side-effects. Thus, the metabolism and immune reactions can be positively influenced, of course not only with children but also in the case of adults. For reason I find it superfluous to mention every illness as there is a Chinese treatment perspective for all illnesses. Therefore I find it superfluous to mention that there is a Chinese treatment perspective for all illnesses. After all, Chinese medicine has been practiced successfully in China for many thousands of years. However, in order to conquer the west it is important to make TCM more understandable. It is not enough to successfully satisfy the health needs of individual patients., If TCM doesn't meet the requirements of the west's scientific, Chinese medicine cannot find its place in the universities.. There are isolated scientific efforts in German universities, not under the auspices of its own professorship chair but dependent on the benevolence of the classical western medicine department. Acupuncture was previously rejected as a method for non-medical healers. Today, however competitiveness has come about because its effectiveness, especially in problem cases or chronic illness has become highly visible and the influx of patients to walk-in acupuncture clinics has become an interesting economic factor. Such clinics on campus could finance themselves and even their own research but also take patients away from other walk-in clinics. Thus, not even endowed professorships can establish themselves in the field of university medicine. At the beginning of the year 2000, the health insurance companies attempted to test the scientific aspects of acupuncture on the back, knee and headaches through so called pilot projects. The tested indications showed clear advantages in acupuncture over western medicine. However, the efficacy of the verum could not be significantly distinguished from the placebo-acupuncture, which could indicate systematic errors. The health insurance companies interpreted the situation such that, if it is irrelevant where one sticks the needle, then the training need not to be so comprehensive and so the fee for this service need, in turn, not to be so high. Scientists disregard the pilot project study on the grounds that there is no significant difference between the verum and placebo acupuncture. Nevertheless, the health insurance companies prevailed in their decision in favour of acupuncture in a "Common Federal Committee of Practitioners and Health Insurance Companies" which decides whether costs for new medical treatments are to be reimbursed by health insurance companies or not. Since 01.01.2007, acupuncture treatments for back or knee pain are covered by health insurance policies. However, because the majority of CHI physicians do not practice acupuncture, they fear that the reimbursement for acupuncture treatment could reduce their own incomes. This leads to internal conflict over fee allocation. Because the acupuncture practitioners are hardly represented in fee negotiations, an unpleasant situation has arisen in which acupuncture is not remunerated cost effectively. Furthermore, the basic conditions with laborious documentation are so unattractive that, above all, the well trained and dedicated acupuncture practitioners can hardly make their services available to social insurance on a steady basis. This is a clear indication that in future only the wealthy will be able to afford acupuncture in Germany in respect to its developing CHI practitioners' system. Acupuncture's claim to establish itself as a traditional medicine as in the past in

China would thereby have failed. Furthermore, the health insurance companies' preparedness to pay for acupuncture only as a treatment for pain stands in the way of an unlimited proliferation. Whoever wishes to have their hay fever, nerve-paralysis or chronic intestinal illness treated with acupuncture has to cover the costs himself. It is becoming more likely that the structure of the insurance system will change. Aside from a minimalistic basic care, every citizen can, according to his wishes and needs, purchase additional modules and thereby be reimbursed for costs such as treatment by a chief physician, private hospital room accommodation, homeopathic treatment, or traditional Chinese medicine. The financing of acupuncture would ensure its development. Maybe then the universities' doors would be a little more open than now.

Culture and Knowledge

Edited by Friedrich G. Wallner

Vol. 1 Friedrich G. Wallner: Structure and Relativity. 2005.

Vol. 2 Kurt Greiner: Therapie der Wissenschaft. Eine Einführung in die Methodik des Konstruktiven Realismus. 2005.

Vol. 3 Daniël Francois Malherbe Strauss: Paradigmen in Mathematik, Physik und Biologie und ihre philosophischen Wurzeln. Ins Deutsche übertragen von Martin J. Jandl. 2005.

Vol. 4 Friedrich G. Wallner: What Practitioners of TCM Should Know. A Philosophical Introduction for Medical Doctors. With a Supplement by *Kelvin Chan*. 2006.

Vol. 5 Kurt Greiner / Friedrich G. Wallner / Martin Gostentschnig (Hrsg.): Verfremdung – Strangification. Multidisziplinäre Beispiele der Anwendung und Fruchtbarkeit einer epistemologischen Methode. 2006.

Vol. 6 Kurt Greiner: Psychoanalytik als Wissenschaft des 21. Jahrhunderts. Ein konstruktivistischer Blick auf Struktur und Reflexionspotential einer polymorphen Kontextualisations-Technik. 2007.

Vol. 7 Kambiz Badie / Maryam Tayefeh Mahmoudi: Strangification: A New Paradigm in Knowledge Processing and Creation. 2007.

Vol. 8 Friedrich G. Wallner: Systemanalyse als Wissenschaftstheorie I: Von der Sprachlichkeit zur Kulturalität. Redigiert von Florian Schmidsberger und Kurt Greiner. 2008.

Vol. 9 Friedrich G. Wallner: Five Lectures on the Foundations of Chinese Medicine. Copyedited by Florian Schmidsberger. 2009.

Vol. 10 Friedrich G. Wallner / Getrude Kubiena / Martin J. Jandel (eds.): Understanding Traditional Chinese Medicine. Consultant: Lena Springer. 2009.

www.peterlang.de

Friedrich G. Wallner

What Practitioners of TCM Should Know
A Philosophical Introduction for Medical Doctors
With a Supplement by Kelvin Chan

Frankfurt am Main, Berlin, Bern, Bruxelles, New York, Oxford, Wien, 2006.
105 pp., 1 fig., 3 tab.
Culture and Knowledge. Edited by Friedrich G. Wallner. Vol. 4
ISBN 978-3-631-54098-5 · pb. € 26.60*

In the last years an increasing interest in TCM has emerged in the Western world. This interest is both practical and theoretical. This book is written for all those with a practical interest in TCM; it gathers texts for those interested in TCM in a philosophical way, but is not loaded with too detailed philosophical information. This book is suitable for practitioners of TCM and for all those who are interested in the structure of TCM and Western medicine.

Contents: Objective and Systemic Medicine · Why Is TCM Scientific? · TCM and Western Medicine. A Comparison in Method and Ontology · Scientific Methodology with Respect to Medicine · Methodological Preconditions of the Comparison between TCM and Western Medicine · Philosophical Practice as Support for Medical Practice · Culturality and Commitment · A New Vision of Science (Revised) · *Kelvin Chan:* Comparing the Differences in the Practice of Traditional Chinese Medicine and Orthodox Medicine

Frankfurt am Main · Berlin · Bern · Bruxelles · New York · Oxford · Wien
Distribution: Verlag Peter Lang AG
Moosstr. 1, CH-2542 Pieterlen
Telefax 00 41 (0) 32 / 376 17 27

*The €-price includes German tax rate
Prices are subject to change without notice
Homepage http://www.peterlang.de